MW01242778

MY STROKE
IN THE FAST LANE

A Journey to Recovery

A MEMOIR

Bonni Brodnick

August Willis Books & Co.
NEW YORK

Cover photo: Rock Point Arch Bridge, Spanning Rouge River & Old Pacific Highway, Route 271, Gold Hill, Jackson County, Oregon

ISBN: 979-8-89145-278-7

Dedicated to my mother,
who gave me life not once, but twice.

Contents

1
Easter Sunday Morning

The day began like any other. I splashed my face four times with cold water, a good-luck ritual. That morning, though, I thought of the pings—little blips of pain in my head that I had felt the night before. They'd been coming on for the past few weeks: brief twitching sensations floating through my brain and vanishing. I hadn't mentioned it to my husband and didn't think to call my doctor. "You can't run to the doctor for every little thing," I told myself.

I dressed quickly, took one last look in the mirror, and changed my shoes to a lower heel. After all, I was only going to pick up my mother. We'd have an early Easter dinner and then I'd drive her back to Westport.

The table was set in a springy, pastel theme. In the middle was a porcelain bunny sitting on a patch of fake grass amidst chocolate eggs and jellybeans. And the night before, I baked a lemon-blueberry cake, taking a short-cut by baking a lemon cake (from a box) and throwing a few handfuls of blueberries into the batter. The cream cheese frosting (made from scratch) would hopefully mask the haste with which I'd put together the cake. A ham was diagonally scored, each diamond studded with a clove, and put under a crown of aluminum foil in the refrigerator. All we needed to do was put it in the oven when I returned.

Something by Verdi was playing in the kitchen. "Good morning, sweetheart," I said.

"Do we have any more milk?" Andrew asked. The carton was near empty after he'd used it for his coffee and a bowl of cereal. He'd saved just enough for my tea, another morning ritual: fill an extra-large teacup with water and a bag of Earl Grey, put it in the microwave for three minutes, take it out, and transfer it to a travel mug.

"I'll get some on my way back," I said as the tea bag splashed onto the counter. I reached for a dishtowel to wipe up the mess. If I could only learn to wake up fifteen minutes earlier, I wouldn't always be in such a rush.

It was one of the first times I was picking up my mother instead of her driving to us. Seeing a new scratch on her car every time we visited her made my brother, sister, and I decide to put the kibosh on Mom's driving. At eighty-six years old, she was vision-impaired, deaf in one ear, the aftermath of a benign brain tumor years ago. If ever—God forbid—she had a major accident and killed someone, my family could not bear the trauma, especially with our son David getting married this year.

As I was leaving, I passed the dining room table and noticed the bowtie on the bunny was askew. I should have cut the ribbon longer. The bowtie was too tight.

"Looks wimpy," I said to Andrew as I kissed him on the cheek. He grabbed me in a full embrace. It felt good to be in his arms.

"See you later," he whispered.

"Stellar" was the word I used to describe my life. My dream project on a documentary film saw us getting accepted into film festivals around the country.

In addition, I have decades of experience in journalism, communications, and media. I started in editorial at Condé Nast Publications and later did media relations for film, television, and Broadway. There was a sidestep into private school communications where I was editor of two academic magazines and received two national awards. I had a weekly column in the local newspaper and wrote a book (*Pound Ridge Past: Remembrances of Our Townsfolk*). My professional days were full.

My marriage had just entered a new zone. Our two children had gone to the same college in upstate New York, which made visiting them on Parent's Day easy. Both were now graduated and on their own. David (twenty-nine), lived in Brooklyn with Libby, his girlfriend of five years. He was in finance, and with a wedding in only eight weeks, on his way to a wonderful life.

Annaclaire was in her second year of medical school in Grenada, which by the way, if you don't want to sound like a rube, is pronounced *"Gren-EY -dah."* *"Gren-AH -dah"* is in Spain.

My husband's practice in real estate law was flourishing. His years of toil had paid off. And we had just downsized from a house in the country, where we lived for twenty-two years while raising the children. A more suburban townhouse, thirty minutes from Manhattan, was now more suitable to our changed lives. We were closer to classical music concerts, ballet, museums, and theatre. Also, no more paying to have leaves raked and the snow plowed.

This is all to say that everything in our lives was finally in its place, personally and professionally. After thirty-one years of marriage, we had mellowed into two Baby Boomers enjoying the ride.

When I got to my mother's apartment building, about half an hour away, the garden in front was awash with color. The daffodils were waning just as the tulips took their cue to flower. I always marveled at how precise were the rhythms of the seasons in the Northeast. It was brilliant when I could master-control the rhythm of blooming in my own garden. Achieving it was always a victory, as if I could actually control life itself.

"Hi, Mom," I said into the lobby phone. "I'm here." I imagined her sitting by the phone for at least an hour, waiting for my buzz.

My mother looked like a movie star in her younger years. She had a beautiful silhouette, great smile, and charmed men wherever we went. I used to hate going to the town supermarket with her because it always took so long. She knew *everyone*, and flirting took us longer. But my mother had a long and happy marriage of thirty-eight years.

Mom was energetic (people called her "Ever-Ready Betty") and she was always up for adventure. Though involvement in her community had slowed in the past years, at one point, she was president of the historical society, the local symphony, and the PTA.

Besides all of this, she was kind, generous, thoughtful, and smart. Another attribute was *quick-thinking*. Even in her advanced years this was not affected.

"Hi, darling," Mom said. "Be right there."

She came down in the elevator and gave me a longer-than-usual hug. "Here, take this."

My mother had filled a small Nordstrom bag with random things she wanted to discuss on the ride home, and from the look of it, we had a lot of ground to cover: an upcoming spring book fair at the library, an opening exhibit at a local museum, some arcane article in *National Geographic*, and various design ideas for kitchen backsplashes in *House Beautiful*.

David's upcoming wedding was our main topic, though. The family was preparing for his mid-June marriage on Martha's Vineyard, where we had a vacation home. Usually, we went up there whenever the children were on holiday break, like Thanksgiving, Christmas/New Year, and mid-winter in February. Everyone in the family shared a few weeks in the early and mid-summer, and we rented it out for August, which helped cover the bills.

In the car, Mom sat up in her seat, her eyes sparkling, ready to discuss or learn about any and all wedding details. I told her about my outfit: the quintessential dress for a June afternoon country wedding. British designer L.K. Bennett created it for just this kind of event. The dress was ivory with blue and yellow flowers draped diagonally from the waist to the shoulder. Shoes, also by L.K. Bennett, matched the dress impeccably: slingbacks with the same blue and yellow flowers printed on the leather (*How do they do that?*). With rhinestones and pearls on the vamp, these très chic, two-inch kitten heels were the perfect height.

"Stunning!" my mother said. This was a word she used a lot whenever we discussed fashion. She worked in merchandising and fashion at well-known department stores and often used this bold one-word adjective with confidence.

"How are the invitations going for the rehearsal dinner?" she asked. Found the perfect design: a "Love"-theme stamp. The delightful mother-daughter wedding banter continued.

Then, only ten minutes into the ride, and from a distance, I heard my mother shriek.

"Bonni!"

I was mesmerized by my right hand shaking on top of the console. The car barreled down the interstate highway at sixty-five miles per hour. My mother began to panic.

"Bonni! Bonni!" She snapped her fingers and waved her arms in front of my face as the car continued swerving in the southbound lane. In the background, I heard my mother scream again.

"Bonni, pull over! Pull over!"

Our speed decreased as my right foot, now out of my control, let up from the gas pedal. My gaze remained fixated on my trembling hand.

My mother rolled down her window, now flailing both arms outside of it. "*Help us!*" No one stopped.

She then reached toward me and made one of the most daring and courageous moves of her life: my mother grabbed the steering wheel and veered hard to the right, sweeping us off the highway. The car bounced a few times off a guardrail before coming to a stop.

We were still in full gear. The holiday traffic streamed past us at a racer pace. Perhaps drivers were in a rush to get to their Easter destinations. But if you saw someone frantically waving both arms out the window and their car colliding against the guardrail on the side of the highway, wouldn't you know that something was wrong?

Two hours after awakening that beautiful spring morning, something changed my life forever. I wasn't lightheaded. I wasn't dizzy. I wasn't nauseous. I didn't say, "Mom, something strange is happening to me. We need to pull over and call 911."

The fact is: I felt nothing. In the United States, I was among the more than 795,000 people a year to suffer a stroke.

2
Looking Down from Above

Emergency treatment works best for stroke victims when administered within the golden time of ninety minutes. It was about six minutes since the onset of symptoms. I was going in and out of consciousness when two young people in their twenties pulled up in front of us to help. They ran out of their car. I didn't think who they might be, why are they running towards us. I sat there, blank-faced, clenching the wheel.

The young man reached into our car and immediately put it in park. He looked at me and saw facial droop. I was staring straight ahead in a stupor. I noticed the young woman's red knit cap and thought how fashionable it looked. I was transfixed by her hair floating in slow motion behind her.

When the ambulance arrived, I didn't hear the sirens. I didn't feel the rescue team grab me from behind the steering wheel. With the passenger side of the car pressed smack against the guardrail, I didn't hear my mother say, "Hey, what about me?" A different person could have just climbed over, but my mother was no longer agile at eighty-six. Her mind, though, was quick. By crashing the car into the side of the highway, she acted fearlessly. Betty saved her daughter's life.

The day that had begun so innocently had now become a

nightmare. I had an out-of-body experience as I watched from above. People quickly pushed the gurney I was lying on into what must have been an emergency room. *Look at their expressions,* I thought. *Why such a panic to get me inside?*

There was a division between my inner spirit and body and what was happening around me. At that moment, I felt closest to my consciousness, the essence of me. A voice inside kept repeating, "Keep going. Be strong."

Finally, my connection broke. I lost grasp of the body below me. Everything turned to a faded gray. And then, blackness.

There are so many "What ifs ..." What if this had happened to me when I was alone? What if it had occurred at a stoplight? Or on a hill or at a busy intersection? What if my mother hadn't steered the car off the highway? I would have died; I would have killed my mother, not to mention the horror of being responsible for other people's injuries or deaths.

We had taken Mom's driver's license away a few weeks before for many reasons. It was due to her mental keenness now, though, that she saved both of our lives.

The first emergency room where I landed needed to know if I was on blood thinners. They couldn't reach Andrew. Of all the days, my husband left his cell phone at home while he was at the gym. I mean, *what if there was an emergency?* Like, *what if I had a stroke* and no one came?

They called my son David, who was jogging in Brooklyn, where he lived. He thought that they were talking about his grandmother and finally put it together: it was his *mother.* "Is she on blood thinners?" one of the doctors in the emergency room asked. He didn't know.

The team needed the information in case of possible bleed out. [Note #1: I wasn't on blood thinners. Note # 2: *Always carry a list of your medications with you.*]

We have a "heart thing" that runs in my family. My father died of a heart attack on the tennis court when he was fifty-eight. According to the person he was playing with, he made a shot, grabbed his chest, and said, "Something is wrong." Those were his last words.

"At least he was doing something he loved," was a comment we heard frequently. It didn't help ease our grieving. And one of my siblings had a heart attack, a stent put in, followed about a year later with triple-bypass surgery.

As for me, I had tachycardia, a condition that makes the heart beat more than one hundred times per minute. (It's the opposite of bradycardia, which is a slow heartbeat.) The electrical signals in the heart's upper chamber misfire and cause the heart to speed up, beating so fast that it can't fill with blood before it contracts. The heart muscles can weaken and become overworked.

Two years earlier, I would often wake up in the middle of the night to a racing heart, as if I was running a marathon in my sleep. I knew my heart needed help.

It turned out I needed cardiac ablation.

This procedure fixes atypical heart rhythms that cause palpitations, rapid heartbeats, or skipped heartbeats, which can be due to abnormal electrical connections. Though these abnormal rhythms, or arrhythmias, often are not dangerous, they can become serious when they affect the heart's ability to pump blood.

My cardiologist explained it this way: "Your heart is like a shooting gallery where untargeted shots are firing off everywhere. By stimulating the heart, we can see the areas that need to be targeted and zapped with cauterization. In your case, the shooting is going off with no aim at all."

The procedure is performed by a cardiac electro physiologist. The groin is cleaned with antiseptic, and a local anesthetic is administered with a tiny needle to numb the area where the catheters are inserted. Small, thin-wired electrodes are placed through a vein in the groin.

The catheters are then guided into your heart using a special type of X-ray called fluoroscopy. Once in the heart, the electrodes measure the heart's electrical signals and are used to stimulate the heart from various locations to try to induce, or start up, the abnormal rhythm. Special software makes a 3-D map of your heart and its electrical system to help your physician pinpoint the abnormal tissue.

Catheters are used to burn, or freeze, these small areas of heart tissue that generate and conduct the abnormal activity. Following the procedure, your heartbeat and blood pressure are monitored continuously for complications.

The ablation treats Supraventricular Tachycardia (SVT), ventricular tachycardia, premature ventricular contractions (PVC), atrial fibrillation, and atrial flutter.

(I was hanging out with the last two.)

The procedure was in mid-October. Post-op, I had slight sensitivity when I leaned on my left side. Otherwise, recovery was easy. Within three days, I was back at work as communications director at a boys' prep school. My heart was now beating as any average person's. I was almost invincible. *Hey, I just had heart surgery and I'm back in a snap. Yes, I feel great!*

But in May, seven months later, I received a call from my cardiologist while driving.

"I'm sorry to tell you this," he said. This is *not* what you want to hear from a doctor.

I immediately turned off the road to hear the rest of his sentence.

"We're not happy with the latest cardiogram. It looks like you'll need to schedule a second ablation."

"Disappointed" and "discouraged" are two words to describe how I felt. Also, "dejected." I hated worrying about my family and how this would impact them. The thought of them trying to distract themselves for hours, a *second* time, in the vast marble and stone cardio waiting room at New York–Presbyterian Weill-Cornell Hospital was unbearable.

I was also worried about myself. What if I didn't survive the procedure? And what if the electro cardiologist drinks too much coffee that morning and has shaky hands? Or something else is wrong with him? Under anesthesia, one is in a state of suspension and vulnerable to anything.

But there was no choice. I had to have a second ablation which, it turned out, was much more invasive than the first. After it, I felt so weak and needed more rest. My entire left side was far more painful. I tried to sleep in a sitting-up position, but the discomfort wouldn't allow for a good night's sleep. So rather than taking only three days to feel back in the swing of things, the second recovery lingered. And not sleeping enough, I soon fell into a deep depression. I felt more vulnerable, and the thought of death, and its finality, haunted me. Not that atrial fibrillation can cause death, but when you have surgeons futzing around with your heart, it's inevitable that dark thoughts surface. Luckily, it being May meant that I could look forward to an all-family vacation on Martha's Vineyard planned for the end of June, going into the Fourth of July. Everyone would go: my siblings, their spouses, children, my mother, the whole crew.

After my brother, sister, and I left for college, my parents packed it in from a Georgian Colonial built in the 1920s in Maplewood, New Jersey. They moved to an apartment overlooking the Sound in Norwalk, Connecticut. Simultaneously came the purchase of the house in Chilmark on the Vineyard.

A Yankee Barn in design, it had a cathedral ceiling in the living room and lofts around the second floor. It was cozy beyond belief and filled with many of the antiques and paintings from Maplewood. The Vineyard was a different home base where we could all meet collectively as the Kogen family, and separately when we scheduled for our own smaller families.

But the timing of this June "all family" vacation couldn't have been worse, and it turned out to be a vacation from hell.

Albeit there were four bedrooms and adequate baths for everyone, there wasn't enough room for the many personalities in the group.

There was one afternoon when everyone wanted to go to the beach. Seven people crammed into my brother's flatbed truck, which we kept on the Vineyard. It was one of the hottest days of summer. "Someone" said she left her beach towel in the house. (Notice I'm not giving any names).

Everyone in the truck waited and waited. It took her forever to get the towel. So, "the person" sitting up front on my right reached over and beeped the horn. In the quiet of the woods, the sound was blasting. It was so embarrassing.

Not to mention how uncomfortable it was to sit that close to anyone, let alone this maniac, at that point in my recovery. The next day, I had a nervous breakdown. No joke. A real one. Several factors led up to it.

Still healing from Ablation #2, I was incredibly weak. I felt like a wounded bird, couldn't sleep well, and the little pocket where the pacemaker was embedded in my chest was still bruised and swollen. I could barely even dress myself.

In addition, I had a new sensitivity: I was trying to grasp and accept that the surgery was *a second effort to strengthen my heart.*

To make things worse, we had lived in our Pound Ridge, New York home for twenty-two years when we decided to put it on the market and see what happened. It sold in about five minutes. During this hopeless vacation, the realtor called to say we had a buyer.

We had *no idea* where we were going to live next. My heart, already feeling so damaged, sunk.

Worst of all, my husband and I had a horrendous argument. To put it mildly: He decided he didn't enjoy spending precious vacation time with my family. (Justified.) There was too much drama and too much going on. Too much togetherness. He had been looking forward to downtime, and this "vacation" was far from it. The tension between us was piercing.

We were finally alone in our bedroom on the second floor when he yelled, "You know what, Bonni? I've had *enough of your fucking family*. Enough of this bullshit over every big and little thing. *I'm out of here!*"

His hand landed on the bureau where an antique China jewelry plate sat. In continued outrage and frustration, he took a swipe. The plate went flying and crashed to the floor. I looked at the shards. To commit suicide, I could run a slice of glass across my wrist and would feel no pain. All the noise would go away. It would be quiet.

Andrew grabbed his suitcase next to the armoire, threw in all his belongings, and stormed out. The cowbells on the back door clattered as he slammed it shut.

From the upstairs window, I watched as he walked down the long dirt road. When the suitcase got stuck on some rocks, I ran downstairs and out of the house.

"Where are you going?" I screamed from the driveway. "Come back!"

"I'm leaving!" he said, hauling his ridiculous suitcase as he turned around. "Get in the car and take me to the ferry."

Not knowing what to do, I got in the car. Andrew drove. To get to the Island from the mainland of Massachusetts takes forty-five minutes. I had no idea, nor did he, of the boat schedule.

There was lots of hysteria and screaming as we drove down-island.

"You can't leave me like this!" I was crazed. Andrew drove fiercely, his eyes straight ahead, not responding.

When we finally reached the ferry in Vineyard Haven, he got out of the car and slammed the door.

I got in the driver's seat, shaking and crying uncontrollably. I wanted to end the voices searing in my brain. *You're so pathetic. You can't handle anything. You should be embarrassed to feel so desperate and alone. Look where you are! People would kill to be on Martha's Vineyard this time of year. What the fuck is WRONG with you??*

I remember learning in therapy that if I ever felt suicidal, I would go to the nearest hospital emergency room.

I drove to Martha's Vineyard Hospital and stayed in the car in the parking lot. I decided I had to call my sister.

She and her husband were the only ones not staying at the house. They had sailed over from Newport a few days before.

"Come stay with us," my sister said. "You can get stronger here. I promise, it will be peaceful on the boat."

Through tears, I said, "It's too late. I need help."

I stepped out of the car and walked into the emergency room.

"I'm suicidal. Please, I need help," I said to the person at the entrance desk. I was overwrought and frantic with emotion.

She then said something I will never forget.

"We're so glad you're here."

Finally, I felt safe. I needed my heart to heal.

My sister called Andrew to tell him I'd checked in to the hospital. Feeling guilty for bringing me to such heightened emotion, especially since I was post-op second ablation, he took the next ferry back to the Island.

When my husband walked through the emergency room door and into my room, I howled an animalistic wail.

Later, I wondered why a man had sat outside my room all night "reading a newspaper." I found out it was a suicide watch.

The following morning, they shipped me via ambulance from the Island to McLean, a psychiatric hospital in Brockton,

Massachusetts. After a few days of group therapy and one-on-one counseling, the doctors determined that my nervous breakdown was circumstantial due to several things, including my heart, my house, and *my life*. I would leave after three nights.

A new friend I met while at McLean, who lived on the Vineyard, was released the same afternoon that I was. The staff was unfazed that it took us hours to coordinate when to leave to take the long cab ride from Brockton to the next ferry departure from Woods Hole.

"The Islander," the boat's name, went through endless fog until we docked in Vineyard Haven. My husband was there onshore, awaiting me with open arms.

We returned to our home now, finally, empty of family. My nervous breakdown scared everyone, and they all scattered. Nothing like a nervous breakdown to do that!

Andrew and I had a quiet and restful vacation. My heart slowly began to heal.

Two years later, my heart—the organ beating in my chest, the thing I thought would be all set after two cardio ablations—threw off a blood clot. That's what caused my stroke.

That's why the emergency room doctors needed to know if I was on a blood thinner. A cranial CT scan confirmed that I didn't have a hemorrhagic stroke, whereby a ruptured blood vessel caused bleeding inside the brain. Once the doctors determined that I'd had an ischemic stroke—one where blood flow through the artery that supplies oxygen-rich blood to the brain becomes blocked—they administered a Tissue Plasminogen Activator (tPA), or clot buster.

The drug was given intravenously by inserting a catheter into a vein in my arm. It is paramount that the tPA be given in the first three hours following the onset of symptoms. This helps

16 | My Stroke in the Fast Lane

it dissolve the clot quickly and restore blood flow to the brain tissue.

It didn't work. I was still in danger of paralysis, speech impairment, loss of memory and reasoning ability, coma, or death.

With time being critical—every minute mattered—they needed to transport me to Yale–New Haven Hospital via ambulance. The doctors there were equipped to do something they had only been doing for two years: the mechanical thrombectomy.

A catheter is woven into my aorta, the main artery in the body. From there, it goes into the carotid artery, which takes blood into the head and neck. They continually advanced and retracted the bulbous tip of this device. It got trickier once they got it in my brain because the arteries make a lot of sharp turns and curves and grow smaller and more delicate. Finally, they reached the brain vessel where the blood clot was located.

Inside the catheter is a small piece of equipment that looks like a thin fishing net on the end of a metal wire. Once the doctors reached the clot, they deployed the instrument and caught it in the net. Once trapped, they pulled the net out of my body with the clot in tow. If intervention was successful, cerebral blood flow is restored almost immediately.

As later explained, reperfusion was achieved after five deployments of the stentreiver. In plain English, it took *five* attempts to trap the clot and get the damn thing out of my head.

My heartbeat ranged between 30-40 beats per minute throughout the procedure. For healthy people, it is around 70. Notes from the attending physician read:

"Patient is critically ill (acute stroke, bradycardia). High risk of neurological deterioration. Respiratory failure requiring mechanical ventilation. Has required 180 minutes of my undivided attention during the past 24 hours for one of the above life-threatening diagnoses. Critical-care interventions have included: medical monitoring, blood pressure management, neurologic monitoring, review and interpretation of neuroimaging studies as well as coordination of care. Stabling exam still with bradycardia, with several four to five-second pauses, and one eight-second pause, between heartbeats."

Andrew was afraid I might end up like his father, Leonard, who also had an ischemic stroke. He was wheelchair-bound and unable to speak for ten years. Leonard could chime in with a bellowing "Happy Birthday" when the occasion arose, but otherwise, he could say only "yes" or "no."

"I couldn't stop thinking about you and, selfishly, what condition we would have you in," Andrew said later. "Would you even live? Would you have brain damage? Be aphasic or paralyzed? Would you be in a wheelchair? Would we have to move from the townhouse with two floors, where we had just moved?"

Meanwhile, my mother and my family gathered in the emergency waiting room. My son and his fiancée came up from Brooklyn. My sister and her husband came up from Princeton. My brother, who now lived in our home on Martha's Vineyard, took the first available ferry. My niece came from college in nearby Rhode Island. The only person missing was Annaclaire, who was studying for final exams at med school in Grenada.

The late-night operation took about four hours. At some point, the doctor asked my husband if I had a living will.

"They were preparing us for the worst," said Andrew. "The rest of the family was there, but I remember looking at David (our son), and our eyes locked. After the doctor spoke to us, we turned to one another and collapsed, sobbing into each other's arms."

After surgery that night, the medical team performed an MRI. In the morning, Dr. David Greer, a professor of neurology at Yale Medical School, was making the rounds with med students.

"He looked at the MRI and said, 'This woman will make an excellent recovery.' That's precisely what he said," my husband recalled. "Dr. Greer also said the first few days after surgery wouldn't be great because there was inflammation around the artery from which they pulled the clot. After that, it would take a few days to see any improvement. "But it felt the world was lifted from my shoulders," my husband continued. "I always say it was the worst day of my life not knowing if you would live, and the best day of my life because you were hanging on."

I had a long way to go to recover, but the verdict was in: I would not only live but would survive and thrive.

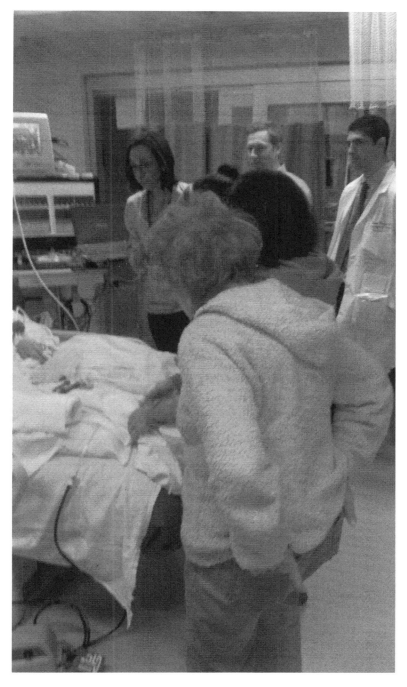

My mother and the medical team surrounding me in ICU

3
Hawaii Day in the ICU

It was seventy-two hours, or three days, post-surgery. I was half-conscious and in a thick morass of fatigue.

The feeding tube strung from the back of my throat to my stomach felt strange. I held back choking when I tried to talk. I gazed around the room. My eyes caught the many flower arrangements on the window shelf. I still had no idea what had happened to me.

Andrew read the message cards attached to each arrangement.

"Good luck! We love you."

"Get well soon!"

"So sorry to hear about your stroke."

This was how I learned I'd had one. The stroke was why doctors and nurses hovered around me, and my family stared at me.

I could feel that I was in an emergency setting. But where? How did I get there? What happened?

"Those are beautiful," I said.

"Listen, she's trying to say something," my dearest son said. "What did you say, Mom?"

"*The flowers.*"

The stroke affected my speech. I spoke in a whisper which was a great way to get everyone's attention, especially when you have center stage with your bed in the middle of the room in the ICU.

I cleared my throat, but the feeding tube got in the way.

"So beautiful," I muttered. Dribble slid down the right side of my mouth. In this sleepy state of consciousness, my body felt heavy. I tried to sit up but I couldn't move. My right arm, glued to my side, hurt terribly. I later learned my mother, who seized the wheel mightily to crash the car, damaged the muscle.

Now I was here, in this critical-care room, where life can hang by a thread. No one wanted to leave me alone. Either my husband, brother, or sister stayed with me in the chair that turned into a bed in the far-left corner. The nurses gave a sheet and cotton blanket to overnight visitors. The patient's comfort was a higher priority than that of the visitor.

And there was my darling Annaclaire. I was overjoyed to see her caring, beautiful face. She had taken the first flight out of Grenada, which had arrived early that morning. Since I was in critical condition, she was allowed to defer her spring semester exams.

I lay there with open eyes. Scared. I realized that something out of my control had happened during that morning drive with my mother. In my slowed-down thinking, I mused on how we can live our lives feeling so organized, and suddenly, something like this happens. Death can jump out at any second.

I gazed about the room. A blur of white med coats closed in and surrounded me. With no strength to move, talk, or think further, I went back to sleep. I slept for hours dreamlessly.

When I awoke, the doctors barraged me with questions. "Can you touch your nose?"

I first tried my right, which I would normally do, but the pain was excruciating. Slowly, I moved my left hand to my nose.

"Do you know where you are?" "What day is it?"

"Who is the president of the United States?"

I had enough wits about me to mutter, "Trumph."

Sounds of machines filled the room. Ringing. Beeping. Buzzing. Bright lights flashed on dark screens as the monitors tracked every movement of my heart and breath. The medical team patiently waited for responses.

My family desperately tried to be upbeat around me. Little did I know that they completely broke down after leaving me to go the waiting room. They were afraid that the stroke might have caused brain damage. Grasping for levity, they decided to have "Hawaii Day in ICU."

After college, Annaclaire had a two-year commitment with Teach for America in Hawaii. We visited her frequently and fell in love with this Polynesian Island, its culture, and its music. The gentle sway of palm trees now seemed so far away.

On this "Special Event Red Letter Day" in the ICU, my husband was in charge of tuning in Spotify to play Hawaiian blues, jazz, classical music, slide guitar, ukuleles, and the otherwise poetic melody that is pure Hawaii. David, in the field of finance during the day and an accomplished ukulele player on the side, brought his uke and lulled me back to sleep with "Over the Rainbow" and "Isle of Aloha."

My daughter tickled my arm, which I always did to the children when they weren't feeling well. And even though I couldn't free myself from the monitors and tubes, stand up, and do the hula, Andrew, David, and Annaclaire could see the music was transporting me.

I dozed intermittently and couldn't think clearly, or stay awake for long. The physical and emotional weakness was profound. But I could feel the love and devotion all around me. Hawaiian music in this ICU setting brought a renewed sense of life and love from my family.

A swath of white-coated doctors stood around with clipboards doing last checks. Finally, they considered me strong enough for the next recovery step: the critical-care unit. Nurses fluttered about as they prepared my departure. When they pulled out the feeding tube, I noticed a splattering of brown liquid fly out of my mouth. In my daze, I couldn't figure out what it was.

My husband thanked the team for all they had done.

It was finally time to empty the room to prepare it for the next neurological emergency. "Recovery," to my doctors, was seeing me able to get out of bed, walk to the bathroom and, if it was a good day, walk in the hall without assistance from the nurses.

I had a long way to go.

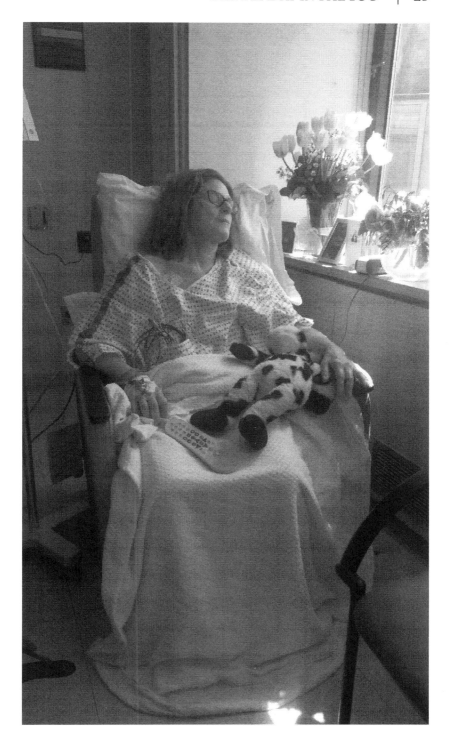

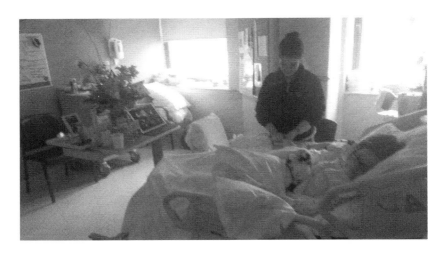

Annaclaire tickling my arm

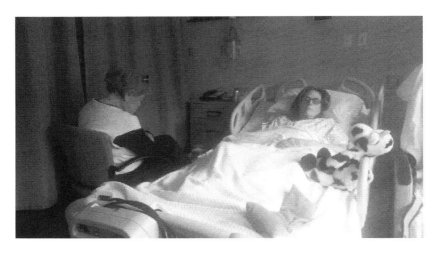

My mother resting while I sleep

4
Make Your Recovery Down the Hall

As the hospital attendant wheeled me through the halls, I stared up and watched the industrial lights on the ceiling pass, one by one. I closed my eyes. The room seemed so far away. When we finally reached the two-bed critical care unit, I was exhausted, and I hadn't done anything but lay there and watch the passing lights.

On the first day in recovery, I was given socks with rubber tractions so I wouldn't fall. "This will help your feet get a steady grip on the floor," one of the nurses said. She also showed me how to wear two hospital gowns to cover up for über-discretion. Wear one with the back open and the second one over that, with the front open. Objective: to get my ass moving but not showing. I should have asked someone to bring me an actual bathrobe from home. It was easier "thought" than "said." I was having trouble talking.

My room had a window. Before I arrived, a nurse had lined up the vases of flowers on my windowsill. The enormous outpouring of support gave me the strength to persevere. It made me proud to have so many friends. By now, get-well cards began to arrive, too. This constant flow of flowers and cards reminded me to stay with it.

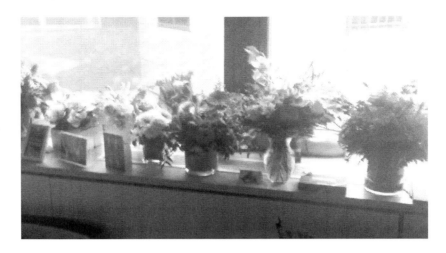

Keep going. Don't give up.

A curtain separated me from the other patient in the room. She said nothing. Not one word. Her family kept talking to her as if she were participating in the conversation. It was so sad.

By the end of the day, they moved in another patient. She groaned all night. I hardly slept.

On the second day, Nancy and Jean, two physical therapists, stopped by. They were fortyish, one slightly taller than the other, and both loved what they did. I lay there in bed, still so wan. Their zealous cheeriness was annoying.

"Good morning," said Jean. She was wearing a loose polar-fleece royal blue jacket with the hospital logo. "Ready to take a walk with us?"

I mumbled. They took it as a "yes."

Nancy leaned over to gently secure me by my upper arms. Jean stood by with her finger on my back in case I tipped over.

Finally, on the count of three, they got me to stand with a walker for support. "Stand straight," said Nancy. I noticed she wore the vest version of Jean's logoed jacket. "Now, take one baby step."

I took a few steps but almost fell over. I was bone exhausted. In hospital speak, "Fall Risk" was my new official label.

"We'll try again tomorrow," Jean said when they returned me to bed. I appreciated how gentle she and Nancy were with me. They mentioned they'd been working as a team for many years. I could tell. They laughed at one another's jokes a lot.

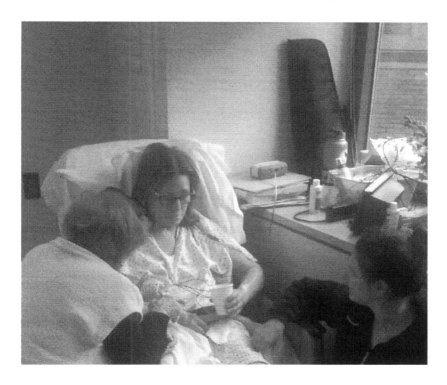

As promised, the next afternoon, Jean and Nancy returned. They switched spots. Jean helped me stand, and Nancy used her finger to steady me.

"Do you think you can walk towards the door? We'll be right here next to you," Jean said as she pointed to the bathroom. It was a million miles away.

"Maybe even make it to the hall," Nancy said. The hall was *two* million miles away.

I took a few steps but was too fragile, and my head swam. I wasn't strong enough to walk to the bathroom, not to mention to the door and down the hall. I needed to rest. Nancy helped me back into bed as Jean straightened the white hospital blanket. It was as if she were tucking me in. Tomorrow, we will try again.

The next day I felt stronger. Jean and Nancy helped me get out of bed and positioned me in front of the walker again. When I slowly stood straight, I didn't get dizzy, just lightheaded.

Very slowly, I took one step and struggled hard to take a second step. I eventually made it past the bathroom, the door, and there it was.

The Hall.

I looked both ways before stepping out. The lights on the ceiling shined bright fluorescent over the surgical machines. Empty beds with complex metal frames lined the walls. I imagined the life-threatening accidents or diseases that had transformed each person into a critical-care patient here.

I decided to take the route that had no obstructions and turned left. My feet shuffled ahead a few steps as I pulled the walker to keep up. Jean and Nancy stood close by to spot me.

"There you go!" they said in unison, encouraging me to go further.

Sure, I wanted to walk further and get the hell on with my life, not to be the focus of attention of my family and friends. I wanted out of the dreary Yale–New Haven Hospital setting and into a life unscathed by a stroke.

With each step, I was gaining strength. I kept saying to myself, *"I can do it. I can do it."* This attitude of perseverance and tenacity would prove helpful throughout my recovery. You don't have to be an athlete, but you must find something physically active that you enjoy doing. You want to be in the top, or near the top, condition (whatever that is for you), so should a stroke happen, there's a little voice inside saying, *"Get up, get up. You can do it!"*

My feet padded lightly, step by step, in the hospital socks. The fatigue was overwhelming, and all I wanted to do was turn around and go to bed. In this post-surgery brain fog, I kept thinking about my immediate family. My children still needed me as a mother. I had to be strong for them, but I was hanging so tenuously to this role.

Andrew was a shining star. I thought about how he could have ditched me when he saw how much trouble I had walking, talking, feeding myself, and just *being*. Yet, he consistently said, "I love you." And "It's my job to take care of you."

By the third day, I could sit up for more extended periods, either in bed or on a hospital chair with pillows to keep me upright. And I was getting steadier on the walker. I could walk to the bathroom, and a nurse was no longer waiting outside to be sure I was okay. To build myself up, I continued unassisted slow walks down the hall. So many people were counting on me to get better.

The pain in my right arm felt like someone was gauging it with a knife and then twisting it. In addition, my right hand started curling during the night, making this quick clench-open, clench-closed spastic motion. My legs felt stiff and uncoordinated.

The stroke must have also affected my optic nerves. Everything looked stretched out. Although I had seen double since I was four years old, now it was different. If someone was talking to me, their jaw was so long it distorted their face cartoonishly. If they only knew why I was staring at them and what I saw: a face reaching down to their chest à là Jim Carrey in *The Mask*.

Acute inpatients had to order their food from the food service three times a day by phone. I had trouble talking, finding the words, and mouthing the words. I even had difficulty raising my voice. The person on the other end of the line invariably couldn't hear me.

"I'm sorry. Could you repeat that?"

I'd try again—even though I was speaking slower and pronouncing each syllable as precisely as possible. Whenever I had visitors, I passed them the menu to take over this irksome task.

Once the food arrived, I stared at it but eventually attempted to eat. It took effort. My throat muscles were weak, and it was a struggle to swallow. In addition, I was used to being right-handed, so I was having trouble getting a forkful of food into my mouth, chewing it, and even keeping it in my mouth because of the slight droop.

Sometimes family or friends helped me eat. They'd hold the fork and bring it closer to my mouth. Every time I took a bite, they'd say, "Good girl," as if I was a dog. Or, "You can't regain your strength if you don't eat." I had already dropped a few pounds I didn't need to lose.

When the weekends rolled around, hospitals had a definite change of rhythm—hours dragged. With limited floor staff, everything ran slower. The doctors and their attending Residency students were behind schedule, and there were no visits from the physical therapists. Nurses still checked my temperature and vitals, but less frequently.

Likewise, breakfast/lunch/dinner ordered from the cafeteria took longer. This slow motion in the hospital cafeteria meant something I called in might have a delicious description on the menu, but after it was delivered, I'd pick up the metal lid only to find the meal cold. It was disheartening.

My sister, daughter, and I watched old movies on the television. One would sit beside me on the bed and the other in the hospital armchair. It bothered me when Pamela or Annaclaire thought something was funny in the film. It felt like they were fake-laughing because they were uncomfortable with me in this new post-stroke state and were trying to break the tension. I was wrong, of course.

The following Monday, I awoke to doctors talking back and forth around my bed. Their conversations were loud and confused me. All I understood was Andrew trying to find an opening at an acute-care inpatient rehab near where we lived. The intensive speech, occupational, and physical therapy programs would help me transition to life at home.

In my half-thinking headspace, I could think of one thing: I was ready to make whatever next steps I could to lead me far away from there.

5
Email Update from My Sister: I'm Beginning to Speak

My sister had begun sending emails to family and friends so they could keep track of my recovery.

Dearest Bonomo lovers,

Thank you so, so much for all of your thoughtful emails.

I left New Haven the other day as Bonni was tenderly looked after by her clan: Andrew, at hand, and David & Libby coming and going. Annaclaire is hovering, sleeping in the hospital, and getting as much of Bonni as possible before she leaves to return to take her spring-term exams at med school in Grenada. Our brother Michael has been a comforting presence, and Betty, the guardian angel who saved Bonni, has also been by her side.

Although alert, Bonni seems to need quiet and healing time these initial days while she adjusts to her new reality. You all know how full-on she is. Being currently sidelined from work on the documentary and all of her other involvements will be difficult for her.

According to Andrew, she aced the speech test yesterday!

Her voice is low and soft. The facts are a little scrambled, but we're confident that will sort out with time.

Bonni will go from Yale–New Haven to an inpatient rehab facility in Westchester. Being the social butterfly she is, I can't imagine she won't want visits once settled.

I am sure Andrew will gratefully embrace the help of all kinds once Bonni gets home. Annaclaire will be back mid-May for the summer, which will be great ... and of course, there is THE WEDDING, an important goal for Bonni to work towards.

Love,
Pamela

6

Transition to Another Hospital

After ten days, I was leaving Yale–New Haven. A bed had finally opened up at one of the facilities.

In preparation for my departure, the nurses swaddled me in white blankets like a baby. Then, two men dressed in black, obviously from the outside world, entered the room. They were the hospital delivery squad assigned to drive me two hours south in an ambulance truck.

I was able to get on their gurney by myself. The men placed one more oatmeal-toned blanket over me, strapped me in, and slowly pushed me through the quiet corridors of the hospital. Once again, I watched the lights on the ceiling go by, one by one. We traversed long hallways with empty beds lined up against the walls, waiting for the sick and dying. Surely, we were in areas of the hospital that weren't on view to the general public.

We took two elevators and finally reached the outdoor loading dock at the back of a building. I imagined this was where hearses came to pick up corpses.

It was the first time I had been outdoors in almost two weeks. It felt good to not only breathe in the fresh air but to simply BREATHE! Inhale. Exhale. I couldn't get enough of it.

The end of April had the wondrous scent of rebirth. My body still felt like it wasn't mine, but I was alive!

The men opened the ambulance's back door, lifted the gurney, and slid me inside. As the driver hopped in the front, the other sat next to me in the back.

My words were few, my voice a whisper when I tried to speak. How could I express I was scared? What would happen to me at the next hospital? What were "they" going to make me do to get better? Would anyone be able to talk *for* me?

My back-of-ambulance mate acted as if we were having a normal conversation. Pleasant and friendly, he tried to make eye contact, but I was distracted. My vision was unfocused and blurry, even with the glasses with the correct prescription my husband brought from home. In addition, the jostling in the back of the ambulance made me sleepy, so I dozed off.

The highway drive from New Haven, Connecticut, to Westchester County, New York, where I lived, went smoothly until I was jolted awake.

"What the hell??" the driver ambulance screamed out. He made a fast swerve when a truck just missed slamming into us.

"Jesus, can you believe that?" said the man in the back with me.

Great. I almost got to set a record and be in another highway accident.

When we arrived at the next hospital, a nurse was waiting for the three of us by the elevator. She led the way to a room down the hall. Now in my new bed, I watched as the men wheeled the empty gurney out the door.

It was a large room with beds lined up across from other beds, like a youth hostel. Patients looked up at me. I was exhausted from the transfer and all I'd been through the past two weeks. I also wondered if I would be able to get any rest with so many people around.

My thoughts were interrupted when another nurse came to interview me.

"Hi, I'm Nurse Dorothea. Can you tell me what brings you here?" My eyes were over-sensitive to colors and shapes; all I could focus on was her pink lipstick. "Oh, my," she responded when I tried to tell her about the accident.

When the interview was complete, Nurse Dorothea handed me a lunch menu from under her clipboard. "To reach Food Services, you dial 5-1-2. You'll be using that number to order all your meals."

I struggled to remember the three numbers as I scanned the menu for comfort food. It seems that that should be a heading in any hospital.

"May I have the grilled cheese sandwich, please?" The person on the other end didn't hear me, and I had to repeat it. I tried to speak up louder. Frustration was all around me.

I hated being a rehab patient and how my body had betrayed me. I couldn't speak my thoughts or even order something as simple as a grilled cheese sandwich. It was as if my tongue got caught between the hard "g" of "grilled" and the soft "s" of "sandwich."

I became an emotional disaster, crying whenever I thought no one could hear or see me. Preparing for the day with everyday tasks was challenging. It was awkward using one hand to splash my face. And forget about my good luck ritual of doing it four times. I was too depressed to think about how my luck had gone way off course that Easter Sunday.

There were constant reminders my life was now so different.

I was issued another walker and, as I had been assessed in the other hospital, was given the "Fall Risk" moniker. Every whiteboard in sight had it written in bold red-magic marker letters.

My room had a window view, convenient for placing all of the flower arrangements friends continued to send. Each delivery made me feel loved. And although the trees were still bare, the earth was awakening to the new season. I desperately tried to hold on to believing spring was a new beginning.

I wondered how it looked from the other side of the window, spying into my room. Beyond the windowsill, one could see a female patient in black yoga pants and a black top. (Patients were encouraged to wear regular clothes.) Physical and occupational therapists walked in and out all day. In the late afternoon, a nurse brought another stack of greeting cards sent to the patient from family and friends. Her expression was one of appreciation.

And every night, without fail, a man visited her. It looked to be her husband. He pulled the curtain for privacy from the other patients in the room. She and her husband snuggled into the hospital bed and watched television. Some crazy British baking show. He looked bored. She looked intrigued. A walker rested next to them, waiting for her to walk him to the room's door leading to the hospital's fifth floor. Before he left every night, she kissed him gently. "See you tomorrow morning?" He always came for a quick visit before going to his office.

And there she was, alone again.

The patient looked down at her legs, feeling as if the walker was restricting her from everything. She grabbed the handles tightly, moved slowly to a chair, took off her glasses, and put them on a tray. A look of frustration and sadness marked her crooked face, and she began to weep.

She slowly got up and parked the walker next to the bed in case she had to use the bathroom at night. It had been a long day.

The patient finally lay down and fell asleep, only to be awakened an hour later by a nurse who wanted to give her meds and take her temperature.

7

Learning with My Left Hand

Every day began at seven o'clock because nurses on the floor knew it would take their patients with strokes and brain injuries at least three hours to get ready. As for me, it took a few minutes to get out of bed, get my bearings, and wait for the dizziness to subside. I stepped behind my walker and headed toward the sink, which was in a corner of the big room.

I had to get used to brushing my teeth and hair with my left hand. The toothbrush usually dragged pathetically across my teeth and there were sections in the back of my head that I couldn't reach with the dinky, plastic hospital comb they gave us.

By now, the three hours for morning reveille were almost over. Now came the "fun" part: ordering breakfast. I was strangely getting more adept at picking up the phone with my left hand. I imagined, and prayed, that the neurons in my brain were beginning to make new pathways.

The menu, divided into sections and categories, needed to be clarified. For example, pick a juice (cranberry, orange, apple), and move to the egg column (scrambled eggs, over-easy). For cereal: hot (oatmeal, cream of wheat) or cold (Special K, Rice Krispies, Raisin Bran, the list was endless). The graphics were jolting—all the words jumbled together. I plowed through.

• • •

There was physical therapy in the morning and occupational therapy in the afternoon, each session about thirty minutes.

Physical therapy took place down the hall from my room. I stood with my walker wondering how they could call this small room with stairs, balls, parallel bars, and massage tables an actual gym.

"Good morning! How are we today?" Joanne, the physical therapist, asked with authority. She stood by the parallel bars to help patients practice steady walking. Joanne appeared to be in her mid-forties and reminded me of Miss Wilson, my gym teacher from junior high school. (It must have been the shorthair and gym combination. My brain made random comparisons as the synapses repaired.)

And in response to her question about how *We* are doing, let's see … *we're* sick of hospitals, *we* know our hair looks weird because *we* can't reach the back of our head, *we're* exhausted from everything everyone is making us do … and did you know you look like a character in a cartoon with an elongated chin that comes to your chest?

I didn't say this, of course. But this was another thing plaguing my recovery: my optic nerve was still whacked out. Everything was double-double vision (as in fingers duplicated in number, so it was as if Joanne had seven fingers on one hand). I was also seeing puffs of floating white patches. Imagine seeing a gym with a blob of fog whenever you move your stance.

"I'm feeling great," I murmured in my new sexy voice. I took a few steps and felt lightheaded but tried to collect myself on the walker. I watched as the three other patients in the "gym" did things they probably did a million times in their past life. "Simple" activities were now so challenging. Tying shoes or getting up and down from a chair topped the list.

"Would you like to try the stairs?" Joanne asked as she

reached over to help steady me. The five or six wooden steps had handrails on both sides.

Here was the drill: Go up the stairs first, turn around, and come down. Best to take it in slow motion. I often had to take a break and have a seat. Rest, and try again.

In a more advanced exercise a week later, Thomas, one of the other physical therapists, walked the halls with me, which he'd loaded with deliberate distractions.

"Follow me," said Thomas, whose name had an accent on the second syllable. ("Good luck remembering it's 'To-MA' and not 'Thomas'!" I thought.) He had placed an anchored string in the middle of the hall. "I'm going to pretend I'm on a tightrope. One foot in front of the other. Now you try it."

As I followed him, I was confused by the bustle. A nurse hurried past me. There was a distracting and formless patch of red on the wall. Upon closer inspection, it was a fire extinguisher. I moved to the side when I saw a group of people walking straight toward me.

I also had to say everything I was doing. All the stimuli overloaded my brain. It was agonizing to do three things simultaneously: seeing, walking, and talking.

"There you go," said Thomas. "There you go!"

I managed not to crash into everyone and everything with my walker. I didn't! Meaning, I did it! I managed to navigate the busy hall with remarkable aplomb.

My brain continued in jetlag mode, and I felt like I had flown to Europe, turned around, and done it again. Then, I did it eight more times. And, moving my left hand still felt cloddish.

Occupational Therapy to the rescue! There were a lot of monotonous exercises I thought I knew how to do, but my body now couldn't. For example, how many times have I gone to and gotten out of bed in my lifetime? I felt pitiful, but I realized this was something I would have to master all over again if I wished to live the rest of my life on my own.

There was a fake bedroom off the larger gym on the first floor. Kathy, the occupational therapist who was so sympathetic to my frustrations, showed me how to get into bed and lie down. Next, we practiced how to get out of bed.

"Roll on your side and use your arm to stabilize," she said patiently. "Get your bearings. Turn your body, and swing down your legs. Have your walker beside you so you don't fall."

A topless car made of metal was on the same floor as the fake bedroom. I learned to open the car door and bend my knees to get inside. Next, I learned how to close the door. And then? I learned how to get out. Easy? *Not.* I had to do it again and again.

There was also a fake kitchen with more tests-of-strength tasks, such as chopping food. Kathy handed me a knife with a prominent right angle for an easier grip. ("Easy to find on Amazon," she said.) Later, using dry peas in a bowl, I practiced spooning soup into my mouth with my right hand. Inevitably, the peas went flying. I was almost glad because I didn't want them near my mouth, knowing other patients had tried the same exercise.

I walked (with my new best friend, the walker) back to my room full of flowers and napped (again). The exhaustion was so intense.

On another day, the goal of the OT exercise was to try and move a set of colored pegs from one side of the board to the other. Sound easy? I kept fumbling with the pegs.

"We'll try again tomorrow," Kathy tried to cheer me on as I practically fell over from fatigue.

I thought, *How the hell can you be so patient? I'm sitting here feeling utterly useless, awkward, and out of it, and you ask me to do it over fifty million times. Can't you see how agonizing this is for me?"*

I slowly picked up a red peg and moved it over to the right. The peg dangled for a few long seconds.

There goes a red one, I thought. *Now, I need to get these green ones and all the rest into the holes.*

"Here, try it this way," Kathy said. She placed her hand on mine. We picked up one peg at a time. One green. One red. One yellow. She took away her hand and let me do it.

Pick up from the left. Move it to the right. What would seem to be an extraordinary length of time felt like, well … an extraordinarily long length of time.

"That's right," encouraged Kathy.

Everything was moving so slowly. Me. My body. My hands. Even the pegs resisted my moving them.

"You have to be patient with yourself," said Kathy. "You're starting to get it!"

But was I? I felt so helpless. I could see myself hovering over the pegboard, but the brain-connect to maneuver the pegs didn't go through to my hands. My weird eyes saw double the number of peg slots as if they were a black and white Escher lithograph. Some of the holes were elliptical instead of circular. My brain felt groggy, like I had just woken up from a nap. Yet, here I was, trying to focus on a task that was nothing more than Kindergarten play. A few months ago, I could have done it in a snap.

"We'll try again tomorrow," Kathy encouraged as I practically fell over the peg project when the session was over. She got my walker from the corner of the room.

I whispered, "Thank you," and returned to my room across the hall. *Across the hall.* It might well have been across an entire football field. Since my stroke, it was strange how everything was in extension mode: inches became feet, and seconds became a millennium. Hands had more fingers. Faces had longer chins. Space and time were my battles to conquer.

8

No Visitors, Please

The colorful flowers on the windowsill cheered me up whenever I returned to my room. They brought me back to the peacefulness of planting and the feeling of dirt on my strong hands. Now I felt so debilitated. I thought back to my garden in Pound Ridge, glorious and flourishing after twenty-two years. Astilbes, lilac bushes—many of the plantings were gifts from Mother's Days.

"Bonni, it would be good for you to let your friends come by and visit," my husband said one evening while visiting me. "They can't wait to see you."

I thought I explained clearly that I wanted family *only* during visiting hours. No friends.

Through the years, I talked to psychotherapists about my occasional depression but "kept face with friends." They were used to seeing an energetic, attractive, and fun Bonni. Having a stroke was different. I was ashamed for them to see me in such a state of weakness and vulnerability.

"Maybe next week," I said softly.

When my family visited, they tried to be supportive and pleasant. They usually sat on my bed and talked, or asked if they could walk me down the hall. I found all of those things annoying but said nothing. I didn't feel like talking or walking down the hall.

"Have you given it any more thought about having friends stop by?" Andrew asked on his next visit. He looked adorable in khakis and a collared shirt.

I finally agreed. "But only inner-circle friends." I had been thinking about the many friends I had in the world. I knew they worried about my health and welfare, but I thought only my closest friends should see me now. I didn't have the energy to withstand other visitors.

Andrew arranged for our two close friends, Mary and Palmer, to see me. Since they lived in Larchmont and were local enough, Andrew thought they would be the perfect first visitors. They were.

That afternoon, I couldn't control my nerves. I awkwardly combed my hair and put on lip gloss with my left hand. As I sat on the bed and waited, I watched how the shadows in my hospital room changed. Winter's daylight savings was almost over, and the days stretched longer.

When Palmer and Mary arrived, we hugged and cried together. They were so happy I had survived the car crash and stroke.

Andrew was right. While recovering, seeing friends—even if you desperately don't want to—is good for morale. It also gives a sense of optimism and impetus to keep going.

So, do everything possible to get stronger: occupational, physical, and speech therapies. And see friends! Give them the opportunity to show their love and support because, wow, do you ever need it, especially with any recovery.

I had to accept that those who love me would take me in any form because they rejoiced that I was alive. I needed to forget about myself for a minute and think of them.

9
The Answer is in the File Cabinet (in Your Brain)

What color is an apple?" asked Carolyn, my speech pathologist, who came to my room twice a week with words and line drawings on file cards.

I could not find the word "red." She finally gave in and told me the answer. We explored other foods and daily life situations. Most were like distant universes I comprehended but couldn't find the words for. I knew I *knew* them; they just didn't come out.

"How about … What is this object?"

She pointed to a spatula and encouraged me with, "It's a …"

"A ffff-ffff," I made the "f" sound. "A flipping thing."

"Right," Carolyn said. "It's a flipping thing or spatula." She broke it into syllables.

"Your mind is a file cabinet. The words *are in there*," she said to encourage me. "You just have to find which file you put them in in your brain."

We tried some more words. Carolyn then plied me with another question from another simple drawing.

"Where are these children sitting?"

I completely froze from frustration. I knew the answer but

couldn't find the right word *again*. And I wasn't thinking about the moment now. As a writer, I love words. I love the challenge and relish finding just the right one. But what had always been a skill was now depleted.

The aftermath of the stroke was both agonizing and frustrating. I felt stupid and defeated. I desperately wanted to relearn to talk, write, and communicate again. My love for words was everything. I listened keenly to their cadence, how they fit together, where they blended, how they might be interchanged, even how they looked on the page. It probably explained why I was a slow reader. I looked for patterns of letters and even counted syllables in some sentences.

I wrote a book, for magazines, television, and had a weekly newspaper column. I was an award-winning communications specialist, a director of communications at one school, and a director of publications at another school. Being unable to "find the right word in the file cabinet in my brain" affected my career and passion.

And it was not only about finding the words. I doubted whether I could type or move the mouse with my lame right hand.

On the next visit to my hospital room, Carolyn asked me to read groups of words to pronounce and use in sentences. Then, she presented more third-grade-like drawings of scenes of people doing regular, everyday activities. For example, what is the guy doing in a backyard wearing a chef's hat, holding a grilling spatula, and standing next to a smoking grill?

Three weeks ago, I could have said, "The guy is in a chef's hat, grilling whatever is on the smoking grill." But now? I couldn't find the BBQ file box.

"The importance of speech is communication, and you want to keep communicating," Carolyn said. "You don't want there to be a long pause. Say, 'I can't think of the word, but it sounds like *blank.*'"

For example, if I couldn't think of the word "flower," say, "It's something which grows in the ground and is appreciated for its beauty and scent."

The official diagnosis came in from my coterie of doctors and therapists: I had mild aphasia.

Aphasia is a disorder that damages portions of the brain responsible for language and communication, including speaking, listening, reading, and writing. It is not damaging to intelligence. When my stroke occurred, a blood clot, or burst vessel, cut off flow to part of my brain. The brain cells died because they weren't receiving their normal blood supply, which carries oxygen and essential nutrients.

Research has shown language and communication abilities can continue to improve for many years and are sometimes accompanied by new activity in brain tissue near the damaged area. This self-repair—or neuroplasticity—is when the brain forms and reorganizes new synaptic connections.

Usually so keenly acute with words, now I couldn't remember how to even verbalize simple concepts. I would try, but then, mid-sentence, there would be a long silence. I couldn't find, put my finger on, or locate that damn file in my brain. My tongue felt heavy. Often, I'd remain silent, afraid of being unable to articulate something.

Often on the phone, I'd try to excuse my slow speech by saying up front, "Please bear with me. I had a stroke."

"It sounds like you're taking your time to select your words. More sophisticated and deliberate," my husband said. To boost me even more, he would add, "And you know what? I'll take 95 percent of Bonni Brodnick any day."

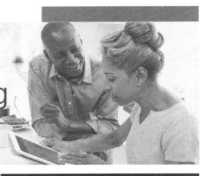

Strategies for communicating

after stroke or brain injury

IF YOU ARE A SURVIVOR OF STROKE OR BRAIN INJURY	IF YOU ARE SPEAKING TO A SURVIVOR OF STROKE OR BRAIN INJURY
1 Take your time speaking. Go at your pace regardless of what anyone else says.	1 Make sure you have the person's attention before you start to speak.
2 Practice conversation first in a quiet, distraction-free environment.	2 Keep your voice at a normal level, unless the person indicates otherwise.
3 As you become more confident, slowly add more conversational partners. Try familiar places like church or neighborhood groups.	3 Reduce communication complexity but be adult. Simplify sentence structure and reduce rate of speech. Don't talk down.
4 When talking to a new person, say "I'm a survivor of (stroke or TBI). Please be patient. Can you understand me?"	4 Minimize background noise (like TV, music, other people.)
5 If someone speaks too fast to you, ask or gesture for them to slow down.	5 Give them time to speak. Resist the urge to finish sentences or offer words.
6 No matter what anyone says, science has shown it's possible to keep recovering! Don't give up!	6 Confirm that you are communicating successfully by using "yes" & "no" questions. Use facial expressions and/or pictures.

The Learning Corp
Constant Therapy

CONTACT US: T 888 233 1399   E support@constanttherapy.com   TLC_MM1044, Rev 1_022019

10

Lavender Shampoo and Living to Dance

I felt a closeness to Kathy, my occupational therapist. Besides doing eye/hand coordination by putting pegs in holes, there was also "The Art of Safe Showering."

We went to the room down the hall explicitly made for re-teaching strokesters, or others recovering from brain injuries, how to manage the once-straightforward elements of bathing: how to use soap, washcloth, shampoo, and towel. And, as I slowly undressed, she saw me in my most vulnerable state: naked, afraid, and post-stroke.

Kathy told me she brought lavender shampoo, especially for me, from home. The scent brought me back to being an art student in Aix-en-Provence, in the south of France, where lavender grows in plentitude, shimmering swaths of purple. One of my French friends weaves lavender wands from fresh stems and satin ribbons. The scent is divine.

Who would guess I would have these recollections while standing in a hospital shower decades later?

"You can take your left hand and scrub your head," Kathy said. She was giving a one-handed lesson in "How to Wash Your Hair." Then when I was finally ready to step out of the shower, Kathy showed me how to do it without risking a fall. "The most important thing is being extra careful. Look around you. Be sure you have something to hold on to at all times."

"Here, take one foot," she said, guiding my leg as I stepped out of the shower. "Place it down like this."

I grabbed the sink, which was right outside the shower. I looked pale, withdrawn, and sad in the industrial-looking mirror above it. My face turned down at the side of my mouth. But I was *happy* I was relearning how to care for myself and was now clean.

I sat down in the chair, which was next to the sink. Kathy took the hairdryer and showed me how to hold it. "Here you go," she said, passing it to my left hand. Though it was my better hand, I was weak and still trying to acclimate to using it for everything.

"You can use your right hand to fluff up your hair," Kathy said as she showed me. I hardly spoke. The whir of the hairdryer overpowered my voice anyway. "There, you're all set. You're beautiful!"

Still sitting, I slowly slipped on my panties and wanted to try the cool new way the nurse suggested for fastening a bra:

- Turn the hooks to the front.
- Latch them.
- Shimmy the bra around.
- Adjust the straps over my shoulders.

Next, I put on my yoga pants, which stuck to my wet legs. My T-shirt went on easier, followed by my sneakers, right and left. That day, I was so proud: I tied perfect bows with the laces.

Kathy walked me as I ambled back to my room. I thought about how I'd had the stroke on April 17 and lost an entire month to two hospitals. It was May now, and the trees were just about to bloom. My son's country wedding was coming up on June 17. How utterly inconvenient of me to have something this devastating happen so close to his momentous day.

The logistics of me walking David down the aisle with a

walker at The Agricultural Hall seemed ridiculous. Were these handicap contraptions even capable of going over grass? What would all our friends and family think when they saw me? After the ceremony, champagne and cocktails would be served on the outdoor porch. Could I drink champagne with my new blood thinner medication? And how would the mother/groom dance go? With a mother in a walker? The wedding now loomed only four weeks away.

"You did great today," Kathy said. "Tomorrow, we'll go back to the pegs. You think you can do it?"

I gave an enthusiastic thumbs-up. I believed I really could do it. I kept saying to myself, *You can do it. You can do it.*" (Being able to tie my shoes gave me incredible confidence.)

Much later, it was dinnertime. I say "much" to make me feel better. It was only five o'clock when I picked up the phone to call in my dinner order.

"Hello, you've reached Food Services. May I have your order, please?"

I still needed help reading the menu because the fonts were stretched and hazy, not to mention the continued distraction of floating white spaces.

"Uhmmm, I'll … have … a … burger, … ginger … ale … and … uhmmm … sliced … peaches, please," I said.

"I'm sorry, but I didn't hear that. Could you please speak a little louder?" I repeated the order.

"It's noted you have salt restrictions. You could substitute the …" The person on the other end of the line went on with a long, drawn-out menu alternative.

"Okay … that's … fine," I said. So, yes, let's go with the low-salt blah-blah. The fact that dining services knew this when I called was reassuring. It seemed the whole hospital was better wired than my own head.

"That will be up in fifteen minutes," she said.

From my seated perch at the foot of the bed, I reached over

to hang up the phone. It was a long stretch. I thought I'd have time to take a quick nap before the feast arrived.

"Just closing my eyes for a bit," I said as if I were speaking to someone.

The meal came up. It tasted bland. Maybe a little more salt?

After dinner, a woman pastor visited my room. She talked softly, asking about my accident and what brought me here. We also talked about how I was doing and what I was looking forward to when I left.

"I'll only have a few weeks until my son's wedding," I said. "All I ask for is to walk David down the aisle and have the mother/groom dance without my walker. I'm living for this day."

The pastor asked what I was wearing to the wedding.

We were talking girl-talk now.

I tried to describe the dress. "It's a summer dress with a splash of flowers up the side." There was a long pause before "splash," but I was unself-conscious about my aphasia. "I even have the jewelry picked out," and I slowly described the gold link bracelet and dangling pearl earrings.

"Lovely! And the shoes?"

I told the pastor they were already in a box in my closet.

"The leather is imprinted with the same print as the dress." I also wanted to say the shoes were stunning, with fanciful rhinestone and pearl flowers on the vamp, but now I couldn't find the words to describe them. She saw the frustration on my face and let it go.

"May I place my hands on your shoulders and bless you?" asked the pastor.

I needed someone to do that. "Yes, please."

"May you have the strength to continue healing and face your upcoming challenges. And may your dreams of walking your son down the aisle and having the mother/groom dance come true."

I began to cry. The pastor held me close in her arms.

"Bonni, you are strong. You will make it to your son's wedding and look fetching to boot."

To boot? Phrases still confused my wounded brain, and I wasn't sure what the boot reference meant. All I could picture in my mind was a cowboy boot kicking something, and I wasn't sure how it connected to anything we were discussing. While scrambling for the correct file cabinet, my brain was in literal mode. These plays on words were temporarily on reset.

I never did see the pastor again. I may have been at a physical or occupational therapy session when she made her next rounds on my floor. Her generous words, though, will never be forgotten.

11
Adieu, Ambien Addiction

Unbeknownst to me, the night before my stroke, I would take my very last Ambien. I'm grateful I had the stroke, if for only one reason: It broke me of my addiction to Ambien. I hadn't slept in fourteen years. Slept naturally, that is.

At the hospital, I was given my prescribed meds: blood thinner, allergy, and anti-depressant. But for obvious reasons, the doctors held off giving me sleeping pills.

Common sleeping pill withdrawal may include symptoms of seizures, insomnia, delirium, confusion, sweating, nausea, vomiting, and anxiety. So, thank you, Yale–New Haven Hospital, for weaning me away from all these possible symptoms.

Little did my dear friend Jo realize that her introducing me to this sleep crutch for one night would last more than a decade.

We met in art school in France. Twenty or so years later, Jo and I were chatting about Jérôme, a mutually close friend related to a larger contingent of friends in France. If you met one, as Jo and I did, you eventually met the whole extended family. They became our French family.

Jérôme was like our cousin. Now with a global corporation, he, his wife, and two children had moved to Belgium. Jérôme was imminently dying of cancer.

"Let's go to Brussels for the weekend," Jo said.

"We have to," I said. "It looks like the end is near."

I hung up and purchased two tickets from New York to Brussels. Jo would meet me at the terminal. It was Tuesday, and I had much to organize between then and Thursday evening.

If Jo and I took the 7:30 p.m. flight from New York, we would arrive at about 2:30 a.m. Add five hours for the time difference, and we'd land early Friday morning. Between the trip and anxiety about seeing our unwell friend, it would be a quick yet exhausting trip for the weekend.

Jo and I landed in Brussels and headed straight to the hotel. (Which, by the way, we considered a great find. It had classic, Old World elegance and was right in the heart of Brussels' historic district.)

After a brief nap, we headed over to see Jérôme and his family. We tried to be cheerful but masked how hard it was to see him devastated by cancer. His bedroom, now on the first floor, was filled with oxygen units.

What was equally sad was watching his two young children, ages four and six, and knowing they would grow up without this remarkable man.

"We should be getting back to the hotel," I said.

"Fine, fine, fine," said Jérôme's wife. She always said it three times during a phone call when I asked how Jérôme was doing. "Sleep well. We look forward to seeing you in the morning."

Back at the hotel that night, the bed was inviting enough: thick down blanket, European shams and neck rolls. But we were too heartbroken and jetlagged. I was beat, and tomorrow was a big day. Brussels was chillier than New York, and we would bundle up Jérôme and try to take him for a stroll in the nearby Sonian Forest, a lush landscape of more than ten thousand acres in Brussels. It would give his devoted wife a little break, and Jo and I thought the fresh air would be good for Jérôme. He was looking forward to the outing enormously.

I knew I had to sleep, but I was over-tired and couldn't stop tossing around in bed.

"Jo, I can't sleep," I finally whispered.

"What?" she muffled from under her blanket in the next bed.

I raised my voice louder. "I said, I can't sleep!"

"Oh, hang on." Jo got up. I could hear her padding to the bathroom in her slippers and digging around in her ditty bag. "Here, take this tonight." Jo handed me a small, oblong pink pill. *"You'll sleep like a pig in a blanket."*

The pill was small enough to swallow without water. As I did so, I looked around the dark room. The bathroom light reflected in a gold sconce on the wall. I kept thinking about our morning walk with Jérôme and fixating on the pigs-in-a-blanket hors d'oeuvre reference. The pill was working. Sleep overcame me.

Before I knew it, it was morning. I woke up refreshed. Adjusting to Europe time was effortless.

Once back in the States, I told my doctor I had trouble sleeping. Even though it was a lie, he prescribed Ambien.

You are supposed to take the pill an hour or so before bedtime. That way, the body has time to ease into sleep. But I always waited until I was in a state of sheer exhaustion. I called it "Hitting the Wall." Insomniacs know the feeling. You stay up so late that you are beyond tired and begin to hallucinate. At that point, my heart would get speedy, and I would start to feel manic. I always waited for that precise moment to take the pill.

After I took it, my limbs went limp. My eyes drooped to half-mast. If I was writing in my journal in bed, the effects of the drug were noticeable. Over the years, many people had frequently complimented my handwriting. Here, what was once distinctive handwriting, with g's that looked exactly like the "g" typed here, turned scribbled and messy. Succinct sentences no longer made sense as I oscillated between Here-and-Now and Dreamland. Finally, the pen dropped out of my hand. I slumped over. I was a drug addict—unable to and unwilling to stop.

I kept my addiction a secret from my husband. The children had no idea why their mother stayed up late every night, sometimes into the morning. I was an insomniac who embraced the thrill of the ride to reaching over-fatigue, then mounting mania, always followed by popping the pink pill.

If a friend spontaneously asked me to spend the night after a late evening, I panicked. I knew I wouldn't fall asleep if I weren't carrying an Ambien. I tried to remember to keep a pill or two, along with lipstick and face powder, in my purse.

I tried to stop many times on my own. "It's only five milligrams," I said to myself. "The minimum dosage. *Right?*" Hell, I could stop anytime I wanted.

The last time I tried was about nine years before my stroke. My son was returning to college after the summer break. I, too wanted to start the new semester clean. I didn't lower the dosage. (It's only five milligrams. Remember?) That night, I would stop my addiction cold. I said good night, but it wasn't a good night. I stayed awake the entire time.

In the morning, my son saw my blank stare. "Are you okay, Mom?" he asked.

"Sure. I was so excited about your leaving for school that I couldn't fall asleep," I said.

My son believed me.

I tried to stop several times by cutting the pill in half. I figured if I took fifty percent of a barbiturate for a few nights, I could easily break my addiction.

I pledged to myself every day I would not stay up late that night. Still, I neurotically tracked how much Ambien was left and diligently called the drugstore for a prescription renewal if the count was getting low. I couldn't risk being out. As you can see, every attempt to stop was a flop. I was in a real spiral.

Every night as I recovered from my stroke, I thought, "Sweet slumber." No more drugs. I would close my eyes, often reviewing things that came up during the day in speech, physical, or occupational therapies. My thinking would get fuzzy, and I was mindful of the sensation of falling asleep. I, literally, felt as if I was falling off the edge. Now, for the first time in a very long time, I was going to sleep, naturally.

When I woke, I felt as fresh as a "pig in a blanket," as Jo called it.

It's almost worth having a stroke for this one reason: I said goodbye to Ambien.

12
A Lifetime to Get Better

It was a new season by the time I left the hospital. Flowers were soon to bloom, and trees were sprouting new, light-green leaves. It was my wish, for this year especially, that spring would take me along for its ride of rebirth and hope.

Andrew parked the car temporarily in the patient pick-up area in front. When he and Annaclaire came to my room, they gathered the get-well cards and vases of flowers. Annaclaire helped put my things—consisting of nothing more than "my civilian clothes," a bathrobe, and pajamas—in a small suitcase.

Once outside, I looked up at my corner, fifth-floor window. I thought of all my progress and the long road ahead. As I walked slowly to the car, Andrew opened the door and helped me with the seat belt.

The drive home made me queasy because everything was going by so fast. "Can you go over the bumps a little slower?" I asked.

When we finally reached home, I needed someone to help me out of the car. I could do it, and it had been a week since I wasn't using the walker, but still I needed an arm for support.

Emotion overcame me when, once again, I realized it was mid-May. It seemed strange how, on Easter Sunday, I'd gone to pick up my mother for what would usually be a quick half-hour ride, but it ended up taking me almost two months.

Annaclaire was now out for summer break from med school, which precisely matched the time I needed her most. For the next five weeks, she fed me high-protein meals and snacks. Annaclaire had read up on nutritional stroke recovery foods to support neurons and synapses in the brain. Selecting the right foods is critical for neuroplasticity and helps the brain reorganize itself by forming new neural connections. So flaxseeds, blueberries, salmon, avocado, and nuts were a big part of my diet.

My daughter also made sure I took two major naps daily: one in the late morning and one in the late afternoon. And although I loved being home, I was scared. I was no longer in a hospital where doctors tracked me and nurses gave me my meds on time. How would I keep up my determination to get stronger if I wanted my recovery to continue?

I didn't have enough physical coordination to drive yet, and the moving white spots and persistent double vision were worrisome. So, Annaclaire ended up driving me everywhere, and I mean *everywhere*. This included weekly trips to my cardiologist, neurologist, neuro-ophthalmologist, speech pathologist, pain management doctor, and clinical cardiac electro physiologist (and since when did I say "my" instead of "the"?), including sessions with physical and occupational therapies twice a week, which I now did as an outpatient.

Of course, my primary physician, or PCP, had to be in the loop with everything. We checked in with her every two weeks. Annaclaire even made sure I was appointed a care coordinator at two medical facilities to ensure I was on course. There was also my regular psychotherapist, whom my daughter insisted I see weekly now instead of the usual once every two weeks.

One day after physical therapy, I hit rock bottom. Unlike the small room (the one they called "the gym") that I used as a hospital inpatient, PT was now in a large room on the hospital's main floor. People with all degrees of palsy tried to walk, throw balls, climb sets of stairs, and pull elastic bands, all while being spotted by a PT with years of training.

As I waited outside the hospital for Annaclaire to pick me up, I could still feel the strain in my muscles from the exercises. Then, finally, I saw the car, which looked much better after the body shop had repaired the scratches and dents from the accident.

I opened the door and slithered into the passenger seat. Struggling with the seat belt, I was embarrassed to ask for her help to buckle it, not to mention I still needed to be driven around. I burst into tears. "How did I get here?" I gasped for air. *"Why did I have to have a stroke? Am I ever going to feel myself again?"* My daughter looked over at me, and her hands dropped from the steering wheel. She leaned across the seat to embrace me.

"Mom, I am not going back to school with you like this," Annaclaire said.

I continued to cry and now felt guilty for doing so: rather than me consoling my daughter, she was comforting me. I had to get used to this new role reversal.

"I am so connected to you," my daughter continued. "When you are sad, I am sad. I can't stand thinking you're at home, all depressed and miserable."

Med school in Grenada was far away, and I didn't want to be a burden. I didn't want her to be unhappy when she thought about me. I was afraid it would distract her from her studies, which often kept her up studying late at night, rising early in the morning to resume where she had left off.

"I'm so sorry, Annie. I'll try not to complain." I wept uncontrollably. "Ugggh, I'm such a mess."

She let go of me and faced the steering wheel. I cried as the car pulled out of the hospital and headed home. I was paranoid that she had had enough of me and decided to try not to be demanding for the rest of the day.

Why had I had the stroke? Random. Just not my luck with the spin of the wheel that morning. The stroke was unplanned, unforeseen, and unexpected. Yes, I had two healed heart ablations, but neither one foreshadowed a possible stroke in the future.

When it happened, I was so content with my life. I felt great, my marriage was cruising along, our children were successful, and I loved working on the documentary film. Everything seemed ideal. I mean, who wouldn't want to jump into my life? Then *boom*, it struck: I couldn't move, talk, swallow, or think.

That's vitally important to realize: Live each day as if something dire awaits you, like a stroke. It can happen at any moment. You never know. You could be driving along the highway, and ...

13
Staying in the Game

"Don't go in there! It's so depressing," I said when Annaclaire offered to go into my closet and help choose something for me to wear.

I was usually so meticulous about changing my wardrobe for the season. But now, it was mid-May and they were filled with black wool sweaters, black wool pants, black shoes, and black boots. I was afraid one more "ask" would overdo it. "Do you think you could help me change over my closet?" I asked meekly.

"Sure, Mom," Annaclaire said patiently. I sat in a chair and directed her to separate the skirts, pants, blouses, and shirts, and pack them up. She took my spring and summer clothes down from the attic and coordinated them in groups by color. Once she completed the task, it was a pleasure to look in my closet.

I so respected my daughter. Her post-college teaching stint on behalf of Teach for America was in Hawaii, making it a key travel destination for Andrew and me the two years Annaclaire was in Oahu. Her assignment was to be a sixth-grade math and science teacher at a military base near Pearl Harbor.

One day, I went to Annaclaire's classroom. Maternal pride overwhelmed me as I watched her standing at the door, welcoming every student with a handshake.

"Hi, (so-and-so)," she said, making sure they made eye contact. If they didn't, she reminded them to. Before the day's lessons began, this was her way of saying, "Welcome. I care about you and what you're doing in my classroom."

One afternoon, Andrew, Annaclaire, and I took a day trip to Waikiki Beach on this vacation. Unfortunately, what should have been a day of sun and fun took a turn for the worse. A protective seawall at Waikiki creates a calm saltwater swimming pool. The only rough waters you'll find are those rolling into this wall. That's where the surfers go to catch the waves, which were consistent on this day. Surfable waves were nearly six feet high, nowhere near the size on the North Shore, where you can find wave heights of over twenty feet.

In front of the wall, non-swimmers mixed with those who could swim. How could I tell? Non-swimmers were clutching their ridiculous floaties in the shape of donuts or unicorns. I wondered how the non-swimmers could think these were safe devices. Would *you* feel safe clinging onto a giant, six-foot inflatable slice of pepperoni pizza?

Before the trip, a friend in New York, who worked for a famous swimsuit designer, gave me this kick-ass, turquoise one-piece. And one of the only reasons I remember wearing this particular suit that day is because there was a parade on Kalakaua Avenue that ran parallel to the beach. A policeman was there directing traffic. I walked up from the beach to watch the parade, thinking about how I would never do that back East; how weird to stand in a bathing suit watching a parade. A young (adorable) guy on a float had yelled out, "Hey, nice bathing suit!"

Walking back to the beach to swim, I noticed an Asian woman coming up for air in the distance. Her father was next to her, apparently screaming for help. I didn't sense they were in immediate danger because I didn't speak Japanese.

But as the father and daughter got closer to me in the water, I put it together: she had taken a donut floatie all the way out to the seawall and didn't know how to swim. She'd fallen off the floatie and was drowning. Her father was pulling her in. Her hair was over her face, and she kept breathing it in as if waterboarding. It was a nightmare.

People on the shore came to help pull her out of the water. She couldn't walk. A crowd began to form around her.

I waded towards the shore and stood there, the water up to my knees. Unable to move or do anything. I panicked and started crying. I'm ashamed that I didn't do something.

Meanwhile, my daughter ran to the young woman, now onshore. She bent down on her knees and said, "Hi, I'm Annaclaire. Can I put my hands on you?"

When I walked out of the water, a man standing nearby said he was calling 911 and ran off.

The point is, even if I was sure he was calling 911 (which he didn't because they never came), I had the responsibility to call myself or get the policeman. I witnessed an emergency and could have made a move to save her. But, instead, I just stood there, frozen and crying.

Annaclaire was still crouched next to the young woman as she recovered. Then, with the help of her family, she slowly got up and walked towards the hotel-lined avenue.

I was awed by my daughter and the authority she showed. Annaclaire was calm and patient. She had shown leadership and sensitivity to her students in the classroom and to this young woman on the beach.

Years later, I was the recipient of her goodness and ability to be organized in a situation. I was certain Annaclaire would bestow this same compassion with her patients when she became a doctor.

In the early days after returning home from the hospital, I wanted to "stay in the game." I had to push myself to meet friends for quick visits, which I'd cap at one hour. Going out to lunch was a whole other mind-trip. I panicked beforehand, considering how long I would have to be talking and how soon before I would become exhausted.

A side distraction was watching my jittery hand during lunch with a friend. I knew the damage in my brain had caused these involuntary tremors, but I still ordered the soup. (What was I thinking?) The soup was flying off my spoon.

"Going in for a sip," I joked. "Everyone, take cover!"

When I awoke each morning, I could consciously decide in which direction to steer my day. Did I want to go left or right? Have a bad day or a great day? Pardon all the puns, but it was a deliberate action to try and keep my hands (even my shaking one) firmly on the wheel to stay in the right lane.

Later, when my husband came home from the office and asked how my day was, I would say, "I had an exemplary day!" Even if I didn't, I would say *I did*. It was too easy to be negative. I had to keep myself motivated and, as a friend called it, "Say *adios* to the inertia of negativity."

If anyone saw me slogging through the day, they would think I was barely on the road to recovery. But optimism fueled my every move. Waking up in the morning to a new day is a miracle. I never wanted to become numb to that fact.

"Do you have a new appreciation for life?" people often ask me.

I answer, "Yes, I do."

To start, I appreciated falling asleep without sleeping pills. I valued that I could brush my hair and teeth with my right hand because it was so hard to do with my left hand for the longest time. And throughout the day, I'd take a moment of appreciation. For example, it still thrills me knowing I tied those flashy bows on my sneakers all by myself.

My aphasia got in the way, but remember, it can be even harder on the person you are talking to. I still needed help finding certain words, but at least I knew where to find the file cabinet: In my brain, right next to the file containing my greatest wishes, which is to stay motivated, to persevere, and be a person with positivity, optimism, and grace. I'd say to myself often, "I know I can do it!" Even if I questioned it, I'd never give in to hopelessness and despair.

.

14
Create a Notebook

When you have a stroke, everything is confusing at first. To simplify, put all your medical information in a notebook. Mine is light blue with white polka dots, and it's a real standout on the shelf, which makes it easier to find.

Purchase dividers to separate the sections:

1. **Discharge Instructions:** Put in all discharge instructions from your hospital stays.

2. **Medications:** Create a list of all medications, dosages, and instructions on when to take them. This list will be helpful to have in your wallet.

   a. Doctors must know, for example, whether you are on blood thinners because of possible bleed-out and adverse drug reactions.

   b. Be sure to date the list at the bottom of the page.

3. **Doctors' Business Cards:** Get business cards from every doctor: primary doctor, cardiologist, neurologist, neuropathologist, speech pathologist, pain management specialist, etc. You'll see a lot of them. Take their cards. You will refer to this section of your notebook often because it seems you see a doctor every day, which you do post-stroke.

4. **Your Physician:** Make your primary care physician, or PCP, "home base" contact. Request they be kept apprised of everything.

5. **Exercise:** You will receive printouts of the exercises recommended for occupational and physical therapies. My home exercise program included picking up coins from a flat surface, finger warmups for writing more clearly, elbow exercises, and for coordination: standing marching, wall squats, hamstring stretch on stairs, and various other upper extremities exercises.

6. **Evaluation Reports:** Keep evaluation reports from your doctors and therapists. They can be encouraging benchmarks to read over and see how much you have improved.

7. **Nutrition:** This section will remind you to eat three high-protein meals and two high-protein snacks daily. Remember, your body is healing. Feed it well.

8. *ZZZZZZzzzzzzzz:* The next tab is for sleep. Prioritize it, just as you're doing with exercising. Embrace that sleeping and napping are essential.

Finally, accept that progress may appear slow. However, by making efforts to take care of your emotional, psychological, and physical health, you are on the road to recovery.

15
The RX Challenge

By now, I was beginning to think more clearly. I was getting used to doing things slower. Simple things, like putting on eye makeup, remained acutely distressing. Another word I could use is *harrowing*. Mascara usually landed on my cheeks, making me look as if I had just stepped away from a car accident, which I technically had.

But every morning, I had another new crippling paranoia. Despite my sister's and daughter's decision to define my new prescription regime, I was still flummoxed. No matter how often they tried to explain or color code it, I still didn't understand when, which, and how many pills to take.

When do I take the blood thinner? What about the statin for high cholesterol? When do I take the allergy pills, and when should I take the ones that make me feel I'm keeping it all together, like my depression pills? It was so confusing. I could rely on the nurses around the clock in the hospital to bring me my meds. They would wheel in their computer and note the date and time they dispensed the pills. Whatever was in the little white pleated cup, I took. No questions. Now that I was home, the process was freestyle and scarier. And what would happen if I missed a pill?

I have always been organized, especially in my career as a

writer and communications specialist. Deadlines never fazed me. Working under pressure was always *de rigueur*. Now, I was self-conscious about how confused and stupid the med routine made me feel and look.

My sister first tried writing it down on paper in big capital letters to simplify the RX regime. Her list carefully delineated what to take and when. She hung it on the mirror in my bathroom. But it didn't mention how frustrating the colors and shapes of the medications were. There were pink, white, yellow, and blue pills in a panoply of hexagon, oval, and round shapes. Forget about capsules, which would often be a psychedelic hallucination of couplets in green, red, blue, and yellow. And what's with nasal sprays? One spritz three times a day. Did that mean three spritzes all at the same time once a day?

I had to take two pills, a blood thinner and a cholesterol reducer, for as long as I lived. That could be a long time. Or not. Depression rumbled in the background. I stopped myself and deliberately tried to re-channel my thinking to be positive.

Because my eyesight had blank floating fields, the list my sister put together, bless her heart, was challenging to read. So, my daughter replaced it with a new one. She has dyslexia, so the colorful "Roadmap to Bonni's Meds" made it easier to tell what time of day or night I took what.

"Mom, there's a handy-dandy pillbox labeled *Monday through Sunday, morning and evening*," Annaclaire encouraged. "You'll see how easy it is."

When we got home from the drugstore, I said I wanted to load the pills into the container myself. But prying open the slats was frustrating. My fingers still needed to be more nimble. The pills fell on the floor as I fumbled with them. If it were a white or green pill falling on my bathroom's light-blue shag floor mat, I could easily find it because of the color contrast. If I dropped a blue pill, I had to shake out the rug on the floor. The medication would surface with a lot of hair and dust.

Equally, the day and night sides of the pillbox were confusing. Finally, though, as if it was some brilliant breakthrough, I broke the code: the blue side was for the sky (day), and the purple (dark) was for the night. That is how I remembered it. Monday through Sunday mornings: take the pills in the blue section. Monday through Sunday evenings: take the pills in the purple section.

It was also frustrating to use my Mac computer with the unwieldy mouse. My husband reconfigured a few things by going into System Preferences and clicking the Mouse option to slow it down. Andrew also got me a new keyboard. It was chunkier and definitely didn't match the sleekness of my computer, but my ring and pinky fingers were still floppy (and I used DELETE a lot).

Although my right hand was slowly getting more strength and coordination, the larger keyboard made it easier to identify and land on the right key rather than two keys at once.

Imagine what it would feel like if you couldn't use one side of your body. Having a new pillbox, using a different computer keyboard, and taming the mouse made me aware I was slowly beginning to heal. But I had to be patient. I was reminded of what my occupational therapist said: *"Not only is it essential for people to be patient with you, but you have to be patient with yourself."*

When I went to my cardiologist for a follow-up visit, my heart still hovered in the low-50 beats-per-minute (bpm) range. Although Eliquis, the blood-thinning medication I was on, would prevent another "episode" (their word, not mine), it wasn't the med to jack up my pulse. That would take something else, and this one had blindsided me.

Now I needed a pacemaker to get my heart to at least 65 bpm. As Sonny and Cher said, "The beat goes on."

16
Oh, To Be Fab Again

My new state of post-stroke made me yearn to be the Before-Bonni—the girl who could wear high-heel Jimmy Choo boots and feel confident and poised (even going downstairs), the girl who could talk smoothly and comprehensively on the phone while coordinating television segments with producers or booking media tours with newspaper and magazine editors. It was hard looking back on the organization skills I must have had when, for example, a friend and I produced an event for five thousand people at South Street Seaport when a famous schooner sailed back into New York harbor from Spain.

I longed for the days of being a young mother. But where did I get the energy to write a book and a weekly newspaper column, while also serving on several town boards, and working full-time in academic communications?

I remembered how packed my days were and how painfully long they seemed now. Just getting up and doing the usual things to prepare for the day—washing my face, brushing my teeth, and combing my hair, all with one hand—was exhausting.

I banned everyone from the kitchen the first night we had a family dinner. I didn't want them to see me struggling. For stability, I leaned on the sink while washing vegetables. Using the knife to slice and chop was a joke. (I should have ordered the right-angle knife from Amazon, as the occupational therapist had recommended.) If I made enough noise, it would cover up how weak I was.

"Isn't it great to hear Mom back in the kitchen again?" I imagined my family saying, thinking/wishing things were back to "normal." But if they only looked around the corner, they would notice things were now so different.

One night, my husband and I were reading in bed. He was deep into some historical book about World War II, his usual fare. I was reading *Vanity Fair* and landed on the "Proust Questionnaire" at the back of the book. I got stuck on one question: *"If you were to die and come back as a person or thing, what do you think it would be?"*

It might as well have read, *"If you came back after the near-death experience of an ischemic stroke while driving on a highway at 65 miles per hour and survived brain surgery, what do you think you would like to be?"*

It got me thinking: I missed being my old fab self.

And, can we return to the absolute sheer luck of me still alive? When the stroke hit, I wasn't alone. I wasn't on a hill. I didn't blast through a red traffic light and hit something or kill someone.

In addition, I didn't have the complications most people experienced post-stroke. Although I was still feeling stroke-y, I didn't have paralysis in parts of my body, and I had working limbs. I wasn't suffering from seizures. I didn't need a wheelchair or a walker. I wasn't using a cane. I wasn't deaf. I had so much to be thankful for and many people to be grateful to.

"Power on, Post-Stroke She-Warrior Survivor!" I said under my breath with renewed resolve.

"Did you say something?" my husband glanced over from what he was reading.

"I just said, *'Power on, Post-Stroke She-Warrior Survivor!'*"

My husband took my right hand, wrapped in the orthosis brace. An occupational therapist suggested this hand/wrist brace with a finger separator to help minimize joint and shoulder pain. It also helped prevent my hand from opening and closing tightly, which it had started to do. I would wake up at night, and it would be flapping this strange "clench, unclench, clench" action.

Andrew kissed the orthosis gently.

My continued quest to "Find Fab-ness" was at the top of my list.

Besides, I, and all of our family and friends, were greatly looking forward to David and Libby's upcoming wedding, which was only weeks away.

17
The BBQ and Rehearsal Dinner

It took real prowess to pack for the wedding. The numerous activities demanded coordinating multiple outfits, shoes, jewelry, and other accessories. First, the barbecue was at the house, followed the next night by the rehearsal dinner at Seafood Shanty, leading up to the wedding at the Agricultural Hall. Organizing entire outfits may sound easy, but it was unbearable for someone still operating with a compromised brain.

As June got closer, my recovery continued. Sheer exhaustion still made me succumb to major naps both morning and afternoon. Although the timbre of my voice was much deeper, my vocal cords were getting healthier. I counted my blessings for the ongoing healing progress.

Our Vineyard house was used for family vacations and special events for forty-three years. Little did we know that one of the first of these gatherings would be my father's funeral. Our family welcomed friends from all over for his burial in Vineyard Haven. Now, my father would have loved knowing my mother, sister, and brother were hosting a barbecue here for his grandson, his bride-to-be, and her family.

All hands were on deck to help with the BBQ setup. My brother, who has a hospitality background, dragged out a picnic table from the basement, put it on the deck, and covered it with a buffalo plaid red gingham tablecloth. Next, Michael arranged all the dishes and loaded them with onions, lettuce, and tomatoes.

"What do you think? Shall we put the posters here?" my mother asked. She was so excited her dream to blow up photos of David and Libby when they were young'uns had worked (and arrived on time). "This way, everyone can see how adorable they were."

I did nothing but sit and watch. Another thing strokes are good for is that you don't have to feel guilty about helping prepare and set up for dinner.

"You go upstairs and rest, Bon," my sister said as she carried out a bowl of Cape Cod Chips. (Little background info: They were made in Hyannis, Massachusetts, a stone's throw from where you take the ferry to the Island.) Pamela could see my right eye was turning in from fatigue. "We'll try to be quiet down here."

Libby's family would soon be arriving. I didn't want them to see me. I felt so physically and emotionally diminished from the woman they'd met at the engagement party her parents had hosted the spring before last. But I couldn't harp on that. Instead, I needed to rechannel and think how lucky I was to be there to enjoy this glorious family barbecue celebrating the union of David and Libby. I may have walked, talked, and acted slower, but this babe was on the Wedding Express!

Months before my stroke, I had reserved a room on the side of the Seafood Shanty facing the water. If it rained, we could pull down the side flaps. But rain or shine, the view was typical Vineyard: sailboats bouncing in Edgartown Harbor and the Chappaquiddick ferry going back and forth.

Annaclaire and I figured out a nautical/beachy table setting. We went to Lucy Vincent Beach in Chilmark that morning to collect sand to embed the candles in tall, cylinder-shaped glass vases. We surrounded the candles with sea glass that we bought at a craft store, and then put shells and starfish on the table.

Although the barbecue included just two families the night before, the rehearsal dinner was more daunting. The gathering was a select group of family, cousins, and friends, and it was my first immersion in a large group since my stroke.

The noise overwhelmed me. People talking, the clink of glasses, and silverware on plates reminded me of the day my occupational therapist at the in-patient hospital brought me to the cafeteria. To test my skills, I'd had to point out where the soda machines were, verbalize how much a burger cost, and show where to recycle. It was a dizzying exercise teaching my brain to separate the clattering sounds amidst the setting.

David and Andrew decided I could make a toast at the rehearsal dinner and not feel pressured to say something at the wedding tomorrow. It initially hurt my feelings, but they were right: saying something short and sweet was all I could handle.

The room went quiet when I stood. Then, in my soft voice, I said, "Andrew and I welcome you to this dinner in honor of David and Libby." That was all I said! Honestly, I think everyone was thrilled to hear me speak.

That I *could* speak.

The menu included lobsters, scallops, fried clams, fried oysters, stuffed mushrooms, New England clam chowder, cornbread, cod, and Key Lime pie. The newly-weds-to-be also chose the cocktails: Dark & Stormys and Sea Breezes.

As everyone imbibed joyfully, the side-flaps, protecting us should it rain, lifted. With the wind picking up, everyone hoped a storm wasn't blowing in.

After this celebratory meal, the four Brodnicks—me, Andrew, David, and Annaclaire—returned up-island. My mother and brother went to stay at a friend's inn down the road.

My sister, her husband, and a niece stayed at a friend's house in Vineyard Haven, which was splendid—old Massachusetts-by-the-sea architecture with weathered grey-shingle siding and overlooking the harbor. We were overwhelmed by the generosity and graciousness of all our friends.

David said he wanted to leave our family home dressed as a groom on his wedding day. And so, the following morning, he did just that.

18

The Perfect Wedding Day

The last time I saw West Tisbury Agricultural Hall was on a wintry January day, only a few months ago. The sun was setting on the barren New England landscape. Our family had been up for Christmas and New Year's, and David and Libby wanted to do a walk-through of their upcoming wedding.

"So, the flute is playing while you come in from here, everyone has a seat, and the ceremony begins," said Libby as she visualized the scenario.

"What if you come in from over there?" said David, pointing in another direction. "Wouldn't that be better?"

They walked it a few times and agreed. It was easy to imagine the nuptial procession in faraway June. It was impossible to imagine, even grasp, that I would have my stroke only two months—to the day—before this big event. So much had transpired in my life—in *everybody's* life—between January and June.

I couldn't fall asleep the night before the wedding. If it were the old days, I would have popped an Ambien to go to sleep, but those days were long gone.

In the morning, Annaclaire and I went to the house in West Tisbury where Libby and her family were staying.

A local hairdresser and makeup artist had set up the dining room table with their accouterments: hairdryers and hair sprays, round brushes, flat brushes, eyelash curlers, palettes of eye shadows, and lipsticks. Being perfectly made-up and coiffed was the objective for the bride, her bridesmaids, the mothers, sisters, and sister-in-law-to-be.

I hardly spoke, self-conscious about my jumbled words. I was uncoordinated when I sat in the chair, my movements stilted, and my body awkward. The stylist put my hair in an elegant bun, with flowers from her garden slipped around it. Still, I couldn't put a face on hiding how discouraged I felt. Once again, I needed to reign in my emotions. "Bonni, think about that Wedding Express you said you were on the other night." It became my mantra. I needed to change from "Stroke Mother" to *"Mother of the Groom."*

Soon, I would see a larger group of family and friends who weren't at the rehearsal dinner—those I hadn't seen since the stroke. I prayed this wouldn't take the spotlight because it was David and Libby's day, not mine.

We arrived at the Agricultural Hall to a flurry of activity. The shucker was setting up his clams and oysters on the front porch. Cornhole and Kan Jam games were ready on the front lawn for the youngsters to play post-ceremony while the grown-ups imbibed in cocktails. An entire pig was roasting over a spit. If I had died when my heartbeat was down to 30 beats per minute, I would have missed so much of this glorious day.

I peeked out from the barn as guests came in and took their seats. It was the exact choreography David and Libby had discussed that January day.

A solo violin began to play Pachelbel's "Canon in D Major."

Andrew and I proceeded on cue from the wedding emcee. My son clasped my hand tightly.

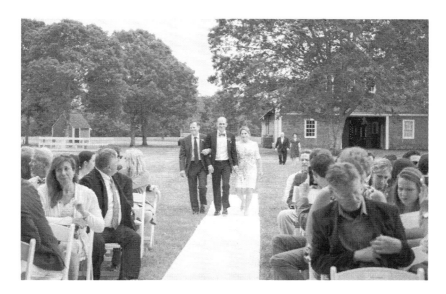

Finally, one of the moments I had lived for during my recovery: To walk David down the aisle. And though the aisle runner lent a regal tone to the ceremony, it was still grass underneath. My husband and son were patient for me and walked slowly. With the news I had had a stroke as recently as Easter Sunday, I imagined most of the one-hundred-fifty guests gathered were shocked even to see me walking.

I reflected on the pastor who came to my room a few weeks ago. "May you have the strength to continue your healing and be strong enough to face your upcoming challenges," she had said. "May your dream come true to walk your son down the aisle on his wedding day. And may you have what you've waited a lifetime: the mother/groom dance."

Andrew and I left our son under the chuppah, the canopy where a couple stands during their ceremony. It represents the new home they will build together. Close friends of David and

Libby made the chuppah and brought it from Brooklyn to Massachusetts.

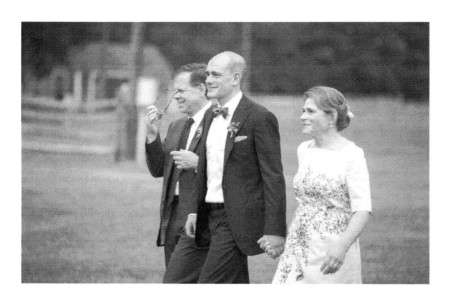

David made sure I was secure enough before giving me over to Andrew. We walked to our front-row seats, as the groom awaited his bride.

When David finally saw Libby walk down the aisle, he lit up. It was incredible for a mother to see this look of such deep love. I felt a moment of great pride and joy, while also the sadness of letting go. We had created a young man who was now ready to take the vow "… from that day forward, for better, for worse, for richer, for poorer, in sickness and in health, to love and to cherish, until death do you part."

Since I had severe double vision, the children thoughtfully chose the shortest Walt Whitman poem for me to read. When the time came to recite it, Andrew squeezed my hand.

I walked up alone and stood next to the chuppah. My hands shook, and I feared I'd have an aphasic moment by tripping over my words. As I nervously looked up, my glance caught Andrew's.

"You can do it," he whispered.

As I stood there, I wanted to take it all in. I was thankful not to have the usual things a person might have post-stroke: a clubbed hand (where the hand is numb and bent towards the body), a limp, or a cane. In fact, it appeared as if *I had been through nothing*. But my gait was different, my voice was softer, and the words came out slower. The audience grew still as family and friends struggled to hear me in the outdoor setting.

"My whole recovery, I dreamed about walking down this aisle without a walker and standing here," I said. "The wedding was my beacon."

Long pause. Deep breath. *Don't lose it,* I said to myself.

"We are all blessed to be here today celebrating the marriage of David and Libby." I quickly shifted to reciting the brief poem to avoid taking attention away from the newlyweds-to-be.

After the ceremony, the bride, groom, and families in various groupings had their photographs taken. Someone was always holding my hand to keep me sure-footed on the grass.

The celebration continued with cocktails and champagne served on the front porch that wrapped around the Agricultural Hall. Children were running around the front lawn playing the games, so well-chosen by somebody in the know of what kids enjoyed. (Libby!)

Later, guests gathered in a circle to watch the new couple have their first dance. Next, the parents took their spin on the dance floor. Andrew held me tightly.

"Can you believe it? You're here," he said.

I always did work well under pressure.

19
Hold On Tight

An exquisite orange and pink early-summer sky set over West Tisbury. From the open barn doors looking in, one could see a crowd of people, young and old, reveling in the festivities. After the first course, the two fathers made speeches, followed by toasts from the groom's best friends.

When they were finished, David walked up to take the microphone. Andrew, Annaclaire, and I joined the other guests who now circled him on the dance floor. Highlight #2 of this evening was about to begin.

"When people go to weddings, they're not just celebrating the love of two people, but the capacity *to* love," said my son. "And I learned how to love from my mother."

I stood there, hardly believing my ears. "Can you repeat it?" I wanted to say so I could relive this moment. "Can you say it even slower?"

I was lost, not knowing what to do next. Finally, David put down the mic and slowly walked toward me.

With an outstretched hand, he took mine.

"Come on, Mom. Let's dance."

What's the phrase? "There wasn't a dry eye in the house."

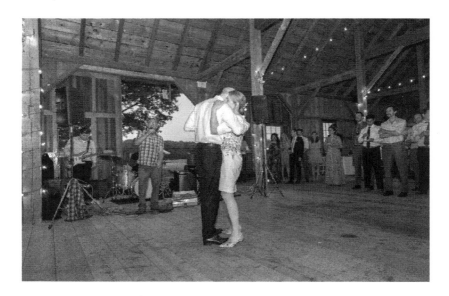

A few months before I had the stroke, I asked David to go over which song we would use for our dance. I wanted to practice it with him and be well-rehearsed.

"I don't want to look like the typical mother and son dancing, where they're stiff and far apart," I had said. Annaclaire put dibs on "What a Wonderful World" by Louis Armstrong for her wedding dance with her father. So I suggested "I Say a Little Prayer for You" by Aretha Franklin or "God Only Knows" by The Beach Boys. We never did decide on which song we'd dance to.

The band began to play "The Way You Look Tonight," the Dorothy Fields/Jerome Kern gem of a song from the movie *Father of the Bride*. Annaclaire and I watched the movie hundreds of times and loved it. "The Way You Look Tonight" was perfect for this sacred dance.

David and I held each other tightly. He had come so close to losing me. I imagined my son's fear when getting the phone call asking if I was on blood thinners and David's panic while driving up to Yale-New Haven Hospital from Brooklyn. And how overjoyed he was when the doctor came out of my surgery to announce that I had an excellent chance for recovery. And what about him playing the ukulele for our Hawaiian Day in ICU? David's unceasing devotion overcame me as we cried in each other's arms.

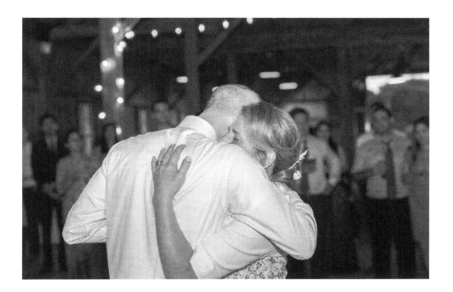

We held tight, never letting go, through to the last bar. David then walked over to his father and sister, who stood close by. They, too, were overcome with emotion. I stood there with my hands on Annaclaire and David, who went to rest his head on my husband's shoulder. Andrew later told me David hadn't done that since he was a little boy. (Did I mention there wasn't a dry eye in the house?)

When it was time for dessert, it wasn't your typical wedding cake. David and Libby went for homemade pies—blueberry, peach, rhubarb and strawberry—from the Scottish Bakehouse.

Everyone was dancing the night away. David's fraternity brothers even sang their school's alma mater. But I was so tired. All my muscles were screaming for bed. The party was still going strong when Andrew and I finally left to go up the road to our place in Chilmark.

Once home, I slipped off my shoes. Except for a few light

scuffs on the sole, they looked as if they'd hardly been worn. Yet, my shoes told a beautiful story:

A mother who had a stroke, with only eight weeks to get stronger, had succeeded in her goals: she walked her son David down the aisle (on grass, no less) and will cherish forever the memory of dancing with him on his wedding day.

20
The Six-Month Dilemma

Now that David and Libby were happily-ever-after and all the wedding euphoria put to rest, it was a big let-down. Something I had lived for had now passed. I knew I had to make an extra effort to keep my focus, do everything I could to continue my recovery, get more strength on my right side, and not fall into depression.

I either picked it up in a doctor's waiting room or was told by a friend that by six months (six months!) the body and mind would heal as much as it was going to.

My neurologist said many people, including doctors, will tell you there is this six-month window of opportunity during the first year after a stroke. I took it to mean whatever you don't accomplish by this mark will be lost forever. If you miss the "window," chances are you will stay the way you are for the rest of your life.

I tried everything possible to speed up the healing process before the October 1st deadline. Maintaining a napping schedule helped me reclaim waned energy. As I slept, I imagined my brain cells repairing themselves and getting stronger.

Since my body was healing, I continued to eat well, including protein at every meal. From my bedroom upstairs, I could I hear the blender whirring and Annaclaire chopping in the kitchen.

My doctor-to-be daughter lectured me on how the body should never be hungry. If it's hungry, it's burning fat, which I didn't need to do. Since April, I had lost weight and body mass, which raised a good question: Why, pre-stroke, did I starve myself to be trim when I already was?

Before the stroke, I usually had a bowl of cereal and a banana for breakfast every Sunday. That was it until dinnertime. Although the calories in this were minimal, it gave me a sense of self-control and empowerment. Since it was a day off from being accountable to clients, I could afford to get absent-minded and spaced out. My husband would beg, "You've got to eat or drink *something*!"

But it wasn't a real fast. A real fast includes hydration with juices or water. Juice, for example, is a food in predigested form. It can be a healthy blood transfusion, filling your blood with enzymes, vitamins, minerals, sugars, and proteins. I drank or ate nothing during my so-called "fast."

I came to learn I had an eating disorder bordering on anorexia. Eating more now post-stroke and never feeling hungry was a game-changer. I was re-learning to respect my body.

Friends would tell me, "You're doing such a great job, Bonni!" Or "You're so inspiring." Their encouragement always motivated me onward.

Upon returning to our home in New York, I noticed something different on the painting at the top of the stairs. When my daughter was young, I gave her a small stuffed mommy bear cradling a baby bear. As I had to stop on the stairs every few steps to catch my breath, and to cheer me on, Annaclaire niched the bears on top of the frame. They were a steady reminder *to keep a positive perspective.*

A significant accomplishment was that I no longer needed the big, clunky keyboard to type. Instead, the slim, chic one that came with my computer was getting more comfortable now that my fingers had become stronger and more dexterous. Even though I still had mild aphasia, when I couldn't find the damn file box where the words were stored in my brain, sentences began to flow easier when I wrote. The synapse between thinking the words and typing them was less deliberate.

So, the six-month dilemma isn't real. *Don't believe it.* Healing from a stroke is a lifelong quest.

By now, I was able to drive short distances. At a nearby hospital, I joined a stroke support group.

People of all ages gathered around a big, rectangular table in a meeting room. Some were more scathed from their strokes than I. Some were in wheelchairs. Some had weakness or paralysis on one side of their face. Some had club hands. Others looked fine until they opened their mouths, and their words were completely incomprehensible. There was an assortment of canes, walkers, and wheelchairs. The group provided a comfort zone for all who experienced brain attack traumas.

After one of the meetings, the woman beside me leaned over and said she needed help getting up from her chair. She had a cane but needed more assistance.

"Excuse me, but can you help me stand up?" I was happy she thought I looked stable enough to support her.

I went for the grab-under-the-arms technique to get her up. It was a mistake. I barely got her out of her seat when I lost my balance, fell, and clumsily tried to grab the table to steady myself. Her cane came flying down in front of my face. At that brief moment, I forgot that I had had a stroke. I had to remember my body worked differently now. I couldn't just lean over and help someone and it felt ridiculous I had even tried.

A comment from an onlooker soothed the awkwardness. "You did that with such grace!"

I also joined a Facebook support group called Female Stroke Survivors. Knowing this group was there gave me a feeling of strength and kinship. One day, I fielded the question, "Did anyone else feel the six-month dilemma whereby they had to be—and would be—ALL BETTER by SIX MONTHS?"

I received the following responses:

"Yes, but I was reminded that recovery takes time," wrote one person.

"No, I don't think there is a set timeline since strokes differ for different people. It's been a year since my stroke, but I still have a left-sided weakness. I may always have it, but I'm able to work and do, basically, anything I want to."

Another person wrote, "Doctors told me the hand is the last thing to come back. They said two years tops. I had my stroke on December 15, and two years later, on January 27, my fingers were moving!"

Other comments included, "With neuroplasticity, if you put in the hard work, you can recover *forever*. I thought I'd be all healed within a year, and now it's almost six! I'm 85 percent recovered."

"It's tough to have 'expectations' and still not be sure what to expect. I'm five years out and still wondering when I'll fully recover." (*Note: This comment ended with five "person-crying" emojis followed by a question mark.)

People say I look fine. "You can hardly tell you've had a stroke," I often hear. But I still have lingering mild aphasia. I try to hide my right-sided weakness, walk with a slight limp that's exaggerated when I'm tired, and my vision now creates ghost images hovering over the solid images. I have to read books and newspapers with a giant magnifying glass because of white gaps in the text.

I can sum it up this way: when I swim, I wear flippers to keep both feet afloat and moving together.

The other day, I was swimming laps at my health club when someone asked if they could share a lane with me.

"I don't think it's a good idea," I said. "I had a stroke and bump into the rope a lot. I think it's best to have this lane to myself."

Be courageous as you rehabilitate. There are times when you feel more alone than ever, but stay strong. Look for live support groups. Join an online group led by professionals, or check your local hospitals.

The American Stroke Association will also connect stroke survivors and their families with a team member who can provide support and helpful information. Their number is 1-888-4-STROKE (1-888-478-7653).

21
Hindered Canoodling

At parties and social gatherings, I was a mess. I was self-conscious about speaking, and my soft voice and aphasia made it tiresome. The thoughts were there; they just took longer to get out into spoken words. Those who didn't know I was a post-stroke survivor might have thought, *"What gives with this chick? Is anybody home?"*

It had been months since Andrew and I were intimate. "The Anti-Clencher" gadget didn't help. Each night, I dutifully slipped my wrist into the bright blue brace, just so, and wrapped the grey felt ties around my arm for an alluring Velcro finish. Picture a negligee. Add the orthosis. Real sexy.

When I was still at the acute inpatient rehab hospital, my husband and I started watching *The Great British Bake-Off*. We snuggled up close to one another in the hospital bed, gawking at the television on the swing arm above us. The amateur bakers went through trials and tribulations every night as they competed to outdo one another with over-the-top culinary creations. I thought the program was a mutual distraction for both of us. (Andrew later told me he hated the show and only watched it because he thought I loved it.)

With the wedding over and having settled into our new and

different life at home, we could try to be more affectionate. But I had to get over being self-conscious about the brace. Even the name of it, "orthosis," creeped me out.

Between the pressures of running his legal office and trying to be lighthearted around me, Andrew also worried about my recovery and how long it would take. As for me, the physical, occupational, and speech exercises I was doing during the day as an outpatient were among the most challenging things I had ever done. Internally, I was also struggling with how I was used to being the person in my household who everyone counted on to show up for everybody else. That role had surely changed.

One night, while lying on my side of the bed, Andrew was reading on his. I reached over to tickle his back.

I shifted my weight until we were spooning. Moving the muscles in my right arm was still aching, despite a pain-reducing cortisone shot I had had earlier that day. And to say it was awkward to have my arm sticking out perpendicular would be putting it mildly. Andrew continued reading.

"Can we trade places?" I asked. He didn't know what I was trying to do but, being a gentleman, he agreed.

From the other side of the bed, I put my arm with the "thing" entirely under my body as if, "Look! Gone! No more stroke!" I reached over with my good arm, but finding a comfortable position was impossible. I finally gave up, completely demoralized, and returned to my side. By now, my arm was smarting from all the contortions.

"Do that thing you did before," Andrew said.

I reached over to try and stroke his back again. Back to square one.

"You mean *this*?" I watched my hand clumsily move up and down."

"That feels nice," my husband said. On the next upswing on his back, he turned over and kissed the bulky brace.

I don't think I could have loved Andrew any more than I

did at that moment. He was racking up reasons every day. And saying, "It's my job to take care of you," was an easy starter.

I'd say Andrew was a keeper.

22

Searching for My Good Samaritans

The elevator doors at the hospital closed behind me. I stood there. Is it left or right for the speech therapy office? As an inpatient a few months ago, the occupational therapist took me on a "field trip" so I would know where to go when I was an out-patient. Why can't I remember?

"You are post-stroke, Bonni," I reminded myself. *"Look how far you've come. You have to be patient with yourself."*

I turned and opened the first door to the left of the elevator bank. It was an office of endocrinology.

"Can you please direct me to the speech and audiology office?" I asked the receptionist. "I know they're on this floor, but I can't find them."

"You're almost there," they said. "Go out and turn right. It's the fourth door on your left."

I found the door: "Speech and Audiology." I could confide in my good friend Susie about my confusion. She had volunteered to take me to my appointments and, during the half-hour rehabilitation sessions, had time to catch up on emails in her car.

Afterward, as Susie drove me home, I looked out the

window. We were silent. My brain hurt from repeating words and scenarios in pictures during speech.

I got lost in a flashback to Easter Sunday morning. I thought of the hundreds of cars driving past us on Interstate 95 at Exit 11. After the crash, I remembered seeing the two people who ran up to our car. I didn't know my mother was screaming, "Call 911!" Or that the vehicle was still in "drive," and they needed to put it in park. There was complete mayhem. And when they last saw me, I looked like a disoriented, middle-aged woman with a drooping face.

Now that I was recovering, I needed to find them and thank them for playing such a big part in saving my life.

"Would you like to come in?" I asked Susie once we were back at the house. She could see from my expression and weakened eyes that I should rest.

"That's okay. Let me take a rain check. I've got a ton of stuff to do," Susie said. "Can I walk you in?"

"No, I'll be fine," and gave a thumb's up. Watching her car go down the drive, I thought about how incredibly appreciative I was for Susie's loyalty and friendship.

To find my good Samaritans, I thought the Darien Ambulance Corp. was the obvious place to start. Before I dialed the number, I got nervous. 'You can do this, Bonni,' I repeated to myself.

Since any ambulance corps treated all incoming calls with urgency, I assured the person on the other end of the line this wasn't an emergency.

"I was wondering if you might be able to help me," I said slowly, pronouncing each word carefully. It was uncomfortable knowing I sounded stroke-y.

I explained how I was in a car accident on April 16 at about 11:30 a.m. when a Darien ambulance came to help.

Could they tell me if they had the name and number of the person who placed the call?

"I'm sorry, but we wouldn't have that on record," the person said. "You might try the State Police and ask them which troop covers that section of I-95."

I hung up and called numerous State of Connecticut troops until I landed the right one: Troop G.

"We're unable to provide this information," the officer said after I explained what I was searching for. "It's confidential."

Another thing embarrassing for post-stroke survivors was crying uncontrollably. The littlest thing would set me off. This time it was frustration. It had taken a lot out of me to call the Darien EMS, not to mention the several tries to even locate Troop G.

The officer may have felt guilty for bringing me to tears.

"Try the Department of Emergency Services and Public Protection. Also, talk with the Division of State Police."

After speaking with several people at the Department of Emergency Services and Division of State Police, I finally landed at the desk for Reports and Records. The woman I spoke with suggested I put my request in a letter. State my name, birth date, and date of the accident.

"Also, include the accident report number," she said. "It will help us track the incident better."

And here's another thing that happens after a stroke: typing a letter. It could be classified as "The Biggest Challenge of the Day." What to do if I will my finger to press a key, and my finger doesn't move? (Which it does occasionally.) Should I forget the whole thing until Andrew comes home and he can type the letter for me?

I persevered. Andrew's lack of patience with me the other night was obvious when I asked him to help me fold clothes. I imagined what it must be like for him, being with someone usually so independent.

About a week later, I received a response to my letter to the Reports and Records department. I was elated! My excitement quickly turned to disappointment, though. The letter in the envelope stated I needed to fill out an enclosed form. The Commissioner of Emergency Services and Public Protection required more information. And to receive any copy of an accident report would cost sixteen dollars.

My handwriting was an uneven and scratchy scrawl. It was illegible. I couldn't read what I wrote, more often than not, and trying to fit the letters into such small spaces was impossible.

Writing out a check for sixteen dollars seemed simple enough. In the past, it had taken seconds; now, it took about five minutes. *Welcome to my new life.*

Several weeks passed. Finally, an envelope with The Commissioner of Emergency Services and Public Protection indicia arrived. Inside was a one-page accident information summary. It mentioned, "Vehicle #1 traveling southbound in the center lane of three lanes on Interstate 95, north of Exit #11 in the town of Darien. Operator #1 suffered a stroke while driving, causing the vehicle to veer into the right shoulder, where it collided with the metal beam guardrail. No injuries were reported as a result of the collision, but Operator #1 was transported to the hospital." (*Note: This is the part that *I love!!*) "Operator #1 is at fault for the collision, and she was issued a verbal warning for being in violation of CGS 14-236; Failure to Drive in Proper Lane."

I was "issued a verbal warning." Seriously? Why didn't I remember the verbal warning I was issued? Could it possibly be because *I was having a stroke?*

I turned over the one-page report, hoping there would be more information, including the name and number of the person(s) who called in the accident. Instead, I found a supervisor's signature and badge number as approving the report. And that was it. Nothing more.

I was utterly despondent. Plus, I was bone-tired. This was surely taking too much out of me.

The next day, I called back the State of Connecticut Department of Emergency Services. Once again, it took several desks before I finally reached the right person.

"Yes, I'm familiar with your story," they said. "It usually takes two weeks to receive this kind of report, but because of your condition, I'll send it to you tomorrow." I thanked her profusely.

About a week later, the second letter arrived. I opened it slowly because I didn't want to be disappointed. Again.

This second report was a complete crash summary report from the Connecticut Uniform Police. It consisted of seven pages of diagrams and numbers. The officer's narrative noted, "… the roadway was dry, traffic was heavy, and it was daylight."

Illustrations showed how the vehicle ran off the highway and hit the guardrail. In addition, there was a diagram of where my mother was seated in the car.

The names of the people who called 911 didn't appear until the final page of the crash report. No phone number, just their names. There they were, Janie and Joe, on the bottom left-hand corner. I was ecstatic. And completely drained.

Every step of this journey in Stroke Land was still so exhausting, but I was determined to contact my rescuers. I couldn't give up now.

To get a telephone listing nowadays, the old-fashioned way, is near impossible and the multi-steps were frustrating. I googled the last name. No dice. Finally, found something on Whitepages.com, but there was the name, no number. I could "unlock" it if I signed up for a five-day trial for membership for one dollar. Sounded like a good deal.

There were two numbers under the last name: a Joe senior and a Joe junior. I called the senior. No answer. Left a message. Called the junior, no answer, left a message. No one was home. After all, it was now New Year's Eve. I remained hopeful the Joe who rescued me would return my call.

Though too drained to amp up reveling for the Times Square ball-drop that evening, saying goodbye to this lousy year was easy.

On New Year's Day, the phone rang at about five o'clock in the afternoon. It was Joe, Jr.

"Hi, this is Joe. The person who stopped on the side of the road for you."

"And my name is Janie," said someone on the line with him. "I'm his girlfriend."

My search was over! Janie and Joe told me how excited they were to hear my voice.

Joe told me his stepmother called him with the news. "Do you remember what happened on Easter Sunday? Well, she called and left her phone number."

After the accident, Janie and Joe desperately called area hospitals to see if there was any information on me. They got nowhere in their search because they didn't know my last name.

"I found the detective on the case and called him to see if I could at least leave my number with him," said Janie. "I wanted to see how you were doing. He said he couldn't give any information out but would give my number to you.

I'm assuming he never did."

No. The detective never did give me their number.

I was eager to learn more about how our lives inexplicably intertwined that Sunday morning.

Janie and Joe were driving home to New Jersey from a friend's wedding on Saturday night in Connecticut. Plus, there had been a breakfast that morning. They were tired from all the festivities and anxious to get home to celebrate Easter with their families.

The couple had been on the road for an hour or so when they saw the traffic starting to slow down about a quarter-mile ahead.

"I was wondering what the heck was going on," Joe said.

They saw my car in the middle lane swerving to the right and a hand waving wildly out of the passenger's window.

"At first, I thought maybe your car stalled, and you didn't have good control of it," Joe continued. "Because you hit the guardrail and bounced off it a few times before the car stopped.

"Janie and I decided to see what happened. When I approached your window, which your mom must have lowered, she was screaming, 'Call 911! Call 911!'"

Joe said he looked at me. I had a blank stare. "Like no one was there. That's when Janie ran back to our car to get her phone and call 911.

"The funny thing was, you were eating a bagel," he continued. "It was in your mouth, and I was like, 'Man, I'm not sticking my finger in there!' Then I thought, 'Yeah, but if she chokes, I'll get it out.'"

As he was talking through the driver's window, he realized our car was still in the drive, so he reached over to me and put it in park.

"I asked your mom what your name was, and she told me 'Bonni.' When I asked you your name, you tried to tell me, but you couldn't talk. I knew you most likely had a stroke because the right side of your face was drooping, and you had no control of the right side of your body. I lifted your arm, and it just dropped.

"You kept trying to nod out, and I kept snapping my fingers and yelling at you to keep you awake. Your mom was saying, 'Get me out of this car!' And I said, 'Ma'am, you're going to have to stay right where you are because you're stuck on the guardrail and I'm not lifting you through that window.' I told her, 'There's way too much traffic. You're going to have to wait until the police get here.'"

Janie explained how she doubted whether my mother could have been able to call 911 herself. She was in shock.

"After we made sure you were okay and in the ambulance, the police took my information, and we were on our way. It was a pretty quiet ride back to New Jersey," Janie said.

"Once my nerves calmed down, I remember thinking, 'Man, I never got her last name," continued Joe. "A few days after, we tried calling the surrounding hospitals, hoping to hear if you were stable. No luck. I thought to myself, that was it. I could only wish you were okay, and honestly, we thought we would never know what happened or hear from you again. It haunted us, not knowing if you made it or not.

"Janie and I are just the kind of people who will stop to help anybody in need, anytime," Joe said. "If it's in front of us, we gotta do what we gotta do."

The following day, Janie posted on her Facebook page:

"April 16th. The day Joe and I will never forget. We were on I-95 coming home from Connecticut, and noticed a car swerving in the middle lane and crashing. NO ONE STOPPED. NO ONE. How could no one stop? It still baffles me to this day.

"Eight months later, Joe's mom receives a phone call from the driver. This woman went out of her way to find us and thank us for SAVING HER LIFE. I am so touched. I hope to meet her again in a not-so-urgent way. Having this woman find us was a great way to start the New Year!"

23
Call the Press

If ever there was a feel-good story, this was it. It was also a perfect example of "If You See Something, Say Something ™."

My mother suggested we publicly acknowledge our first responders' courage. I was a media relations specialist in the past, so I knew the drill for working with reporters, editors, or producers to get coverage on a story.

I asked Janie what her local paper was, and she told me it was *The Daily Journal*. I would use my press agent skills to pitch this inspiring story.

After researching the newsroom contacts online, I tried to identify which reporter might be interested. I called the regional editor, left a message on voicemail, hit playback. Hit erase. Tried it again.

Left a second message. Hit playback. Hit erase. My diminished speech and motor skills were blatant. I talked so slowly. E-nun-ci-at-ing every syllable. It was like the chasm between my inner self and outer being. On the inside, I was gung-ho. On the outside, frustrations abound.

I left a third message and played it back. I wanted to erase it and try again, but that was it. I hung up, frustrated and discouraged.

A few days later, I received an email from the reporter. "Thank you for sending this story idea. It's terrific. I'll be forwarding the information to someone who will respond to you shortly."

When I finally connected (live!) with the reporter on the telephone, she exclaimed, "How did you know I *love* doing stories like this?"

I emailed Janie and Joe to set up a mutually convenient time for the reporter and photographer to go over and meet them at their home. The reporter would also interview me, but I wanted to be sure I wasn't the story's highlight. It was Janie and Joe who deserved the acclaim.

Weeks later, "SOUTH JERSEY MOTORISTS HELP DRIVER WHO SUFFERED STROKE: Couple hailed as lifesavers" appeared a week later in *The Daily Journal* on the *front page, above the fold*. (Prime real estate in any newspaper.) I was so pleased that the editorial team deemed this an important enough story to grab the headline.

After reading the piece, I learned more about Janie and Joe. She was twenty-three and worked as an emergency veterinary technician at a local veterinary hospital. Joe was twenty-seven and worked as a head diesel mechanic at a local diesel shop.

Later that day, Janie sent me this text:

"My cousin, a manager at a local store, was putting the paper out that morning and saw my face on the front page. He texted and told me to check it out! I was waking up for work, so it didn't click right away. Then my friends started to text me. On my break from work, I went to a local convenience store to pick up the paper. Wasn't expecting to be on the front page!"

Joe was at work and didn't know right away when the story would run. "When he found out, Joe was shocked, too. His clients were calling to tell him about it. So, Joe's stepmom rushed out to grab a copy. She cut it out, put it in a frame, and hung it on the wall! Lol."

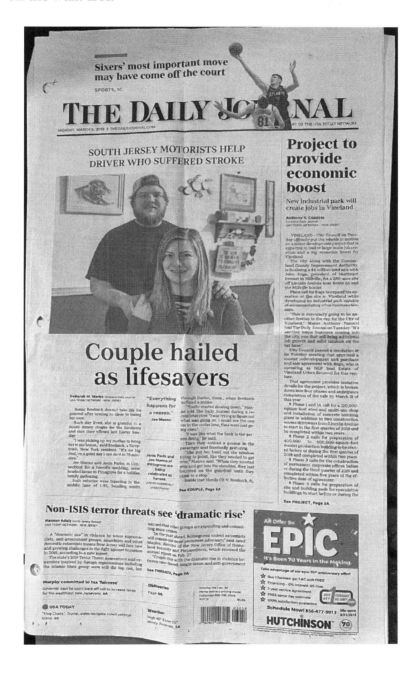

The story ran on the *Associated Press* wire, meaning it would reach far beyond *The Daily Journal* readership in southern New Jersey.

Some of the outlets in which the story appeared were the *Chicago Tribune*, *U.S. News & World Report*, The *Washington Times*, *Philadelphia Enquirer*, *Miami Herald*, *Lexington Herald-Leader*, and *The Wichita Eagle*.

Janie wrote on Facebook, "And the story keeps going!! My mom's friend has a sister in Arizona, and we were on the front page of their local paper. I also found out the story was in Seattle and California!"

I was happy Janie and Joe received national recognition for their bravery and heroism. I hope this story will inspire others to stop and help if they see something is wrong.

A few weeks later, I was in an art gallery talking with the artist. I told her my story and how I could still feel remnants of the stroke.

A person looking at a nearby painting overheard our conversation. She walked over and said, "Wait … I think I read about you. Are you the person who had a stroke on I-95, and some good Samaritans stopped to help?"

Indeed, I am.

24
My Mother, My Savior

Before the accident, my brother, sister, and I told Mom her driving days were over. We'd find fresh dents on the car every time we visited her. My mother also needed more and more pillows to sit high enough to see over the dashboard.

Things began to rack up one night after a bad ice storm. My mother said she wanted to bring over soup. We lived in the country, and the roads were treacherous. I forbade her to get in the car. Unfortunately, she did. She also crashed into a fence at a bend in the road, nearly driving into a lake.

There was a knock on the front door. We couldn't imagine who it could be on such a stormy night. It was my mother, standing next to a police officer. She handed me a casserole with soup, the outside of which was dripping with kernels of corn.

The whole family was afraid of her getting into a major car accident. What if she injured a baby or a child with their entire lives ahead of them? What if *she* was the fatality in the accident? Andrew and I told her emphatically, that we couldn't bear the thought of something like this happening the year David was getting married. It would be unfair to all of us.

Shortly after that, on a visit to my mother, my husband and I saw another gash in the side of her car. When Andrew and I asked what happened, she said, "I don't know. I turned, and there was a landscape truck right there. It was hard to tell what it was. So, I really don't know how that happened."

The next dent, the next alibi: "I was driving under the tunnel by the railroad station, and this car was coming towards me," my mom said, trying to explain why the steering wheel was stuck in this strange angle that made it impossible to steer. "All of a sudden, I had to move over. The car bolted up the side wall, but it was only a little bit."

Bye-bye, car!!! On behalf of my siblings and the whole family, we were thrilled to be wiping our hands of a possible homicide in the making.

That afternoon, my husband and I drove to the mechanic's to finally get rid of the car. "It's all yours, Hordy," I said as we handed over the keys. My parents had been using him for more than forty years, his name even finding a place in family folklore. Hordy confided how he had just replaced a front light bulb, and, in full conscience, he couldn't do it again and feel right about Mom catapulting out of the garage towards the next accident.

My mother was slow to forgive the family, but we almost felt like we were saving society by preventing her from driving. Still, she longingly wished to be behind the wheel again. (I later found out she once asked her caregiver if she could drive around her apartment parking lot.)

Here we had thought our mother might kill someone if she continued driving. Little could we know, in a few months, Mom's quick thinking and sheer fearlessness would make her a true hero on that near-fatal day of my stroke. And, let's face it, without Mom in the car, I wouldn't be here writing this. In that split second, she saved both of our lives and possibly the lives of others around us.

Now I wondered: *What was it like to be sitting next to me in the passenger seat on that Easter morning?* I had tried to ask my mother, but she always responded, "Can we do it later?"

I knew it wouldn't be easy to recount the episode. On a subsequent visit, I invited Mom to the beach, down the street from her apartment. I would record the interview on my iPhone and suggested she pretend I wasn't her daughter. I would have on my journalist hat.

"How about we sit over there?" I slowed down the car and pointed to a bench on the point. "Is that good?"

"Fine," my mom said. A single word. I could tell she was already getting nervous.

I pulled into a parking space. After putting the car in park, I got out, walked over to my mother's side, and opened the door. I held her elbow. She was frailer now, and her cane hardly gave enough steadiness in the sand and blustery wind.

We sat down on the bench: Mother and Daughter. It was a poignant moment for both of us as she finally recounted her story.

"It was such a nice morning," my mother began. "We had stopped for coffee and bagels to eat in the car. Just ten minutes into the ride, we were almost at Darien. I asked you a question, but you weren't responding. You were transfixed. You just wouldn't let go. I waved my left arm before you, and there was no response. I kept saying, 'Bonni! Bonni!' You kept staring ahead as the car propelled forward. I remember hearing myself scream, 'Oh, my God! Oh, my God!'"

"I thought, 'We've got a problem here.' It was a holiday Sunday, so there was traffic. But I assessed the situation real fast. I thought, 'I've got to stop this car.' So, I looked to my right and waited for a break in the cars. When it finally came, I pulled the wheel over as hard as I could and we crashed.

"I just sat there in shock," she continued. "A lovely young couple stopped in front of us and ran over to the car. I said, 'Quick, call an ambulance!' And I must have blacked out.

"When I came to, I was trapped. My door was locked against the guardrail. I looked to the left, where an ambulance had already arrived, lights flashing. Two paramedics were pushing you on a gurney into the back of it. I screamed out, 'Hey, wait for me!' Everyone ignored the old lady jammed in the car.

"I had to climb over the console, which wasn't easy for me at my age. I got into the ambulance and sat next to the medic in the back. I held your hand. With the siren roaring, we drove to Stamford Hospital.

"Thank God they were working on you. I was standing in the guest area alone. No nurse or medical team paid attention to me, which didn't bother me. It was like I was there, but not there. I wasn't a participant. I was a spectator.

"You were the prime concern, and I wanted to ensure you got the best care. I suddenly thought, 'I've got to call Andrew.' I wasn't thinking clearly and still didn't know exactly what was wrong with you, whether it was a stroke or a seizure of some sort, I didn't know. It was all so dramatic. I put everything into action. Let's put it this way: I don't panic. I move into solutions. Get help. Get her to the hospital. Get moving.

"A doctor at Stamford Hospital sized up the situation in about half an hour. She decided to ship you up to Yale– New Haven Hospital. I don't remember how I got there.

"Everybody in the family rallied. Andrew was soon there. David and Libby were there. Michael (who was living on Martha's Vineyard) later said Andrew told him, 'Something happened to Bonni. You have to take the next boat,' and he came immediately. Pamela and (her husband) Michael came up from Princeton. Your niece Rebecca was there, and Annaclaire took an immediate flight from Grenada. You were surrounded by love and by family.

"I remember thinking, 'Bonni is a stubborn kid. If there's any time we need her stubbornness, this is it.'

"I was so happy we got you to the right place. About a week later, you were sitting with Andrew. You were responsive and slowly on your way to recovery. I was so relieved. The worst was over. Knowing how determined you are, it was just a question of time until you were back."

Along with the motivation to attend my son's wedding, the other thing that carried me through was my mother's positive attitude. She attributed much of her inner strength to my father's encouragement after she had a benign brain tumor at the age of forty-five. The surgery to remove it had paralyzed half of her face and down through her neck. Still, she powered on.

A squall-like wind was creating white caps on the water. After a brief pause, my mother continued. "So, after you've attended to the immediate concerns—like getting you to the right hospital and them doing what was necessary to get you better—you get back on the path and forget it. It's over. Jump back into life. That's what I tried to do when I had the brain tumor. I had to set an example for my wonderful children. You don't throw in the towel. You mend the situation and move on. Don't wallow in your problems."

We discussed Janie and Joe. Why did they stop to help us? It was a miracle.

"One has to be supportive of even a stranger," my mom said. "Do what you can to help people. The expression, 'Do unto others as you would have them do unto you,' rings true. I can't recall a single time I've helped someone hoping they would do the same for me. Being kind and concerned is just a part of my nature. It's either in you, or it's not. And if it's not, you should force yourself to be as kind and concerned as you can, whether your efforts are rewarded or not."

I turned off the voice memo app on my iPhone, our conversation now recorded. My mother and I stared out at Long Island Sound. The gusting wind had eased, and the water was now calm.

I was overcome with love and gratitude as I took her hand. She'd survived a brain tumor, and I'd survived a stroke.

"To us!" I said. "Survivors."

I am proud to call this magnificent, courageous, and brave person my mother, to whom I owe *everything*.

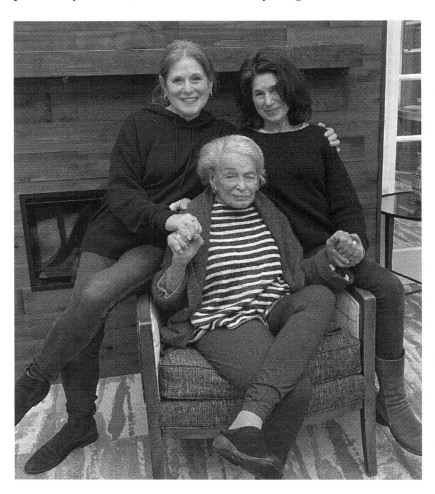

The Heroic Betty, surrounded by her daughters,
Bonni (left) and Pamela (right).

25
Pourquoi PAS *Moi*? (Why *NOT* Me?)

The day I had my stroke began like any other day. Though feeling nothing amiss the morning of this life-changing event, death was a heartbeat away.

I arrived at both hospitals in critical condition. The whole time, I was bradycardic with a heartbeat in the 30s-40s, with eight-second pauses between beats. I was teetering between life and death. The accident caused my words to vanish and my thoughts to become confused. But since waking up in the ICU, I've felt determined to tell my story. I had to find the strength to voice what happened after a blood clot impaired my body and brain.

Through hell or high water, by fair means or foul, by hook or by crook, whatever the phrase in my scrambled head, I would reveal and explain to readers what it was like not to be able to think, walk, swallow, or talk.

It's easy to say, "Why me?" but I think, "Why *not* me?" Why *not* make something like this happen to a person who has just hit a new stride with her marriage, motherhood, and career? It's not that I deserved what happened; it was simply random.

And the truth is: *This story could happen to you.*

It was as if I had tightrope-walked on the edge of a razor

blade. Being so close to finality taught me to focus on what matters most: love and encouragement from family and friends.

Every day I feel as if anyone could tell by how I'm talking and walking that I had a stroke. Physically, there is the aftermath: The extreme pain in my right arm is much better but right-side weakness endures. My vision remains double and always will. My hand has a tremor when I write. I can't swim with the same gusto because my right foot drags. The mild aphasia stilting my conversation is improving.

Sometimes, I can't think of a word, and my mind blanks out. I silently struggle, waiting for the word to come to me. (When this happens, I usually put my palms together in "Namaste" and hum. It lightens the moment not only for me but for others as well.)

My good friend F.P. wrote that she was awed by my recent successes. "Your achievements, perseverance, and the goals you have set for yourself—relearning many basic tasks, to a mother/son dance, to writing your story. All just an amazing and magical journey and testament to your incredible inner strength."

This inner strength doesn't always work together as smoothly with the awkwardness I often feel with my outer physical being. Yet, a renewed sense of self empowers me. I push myself when exercising and take my time when walking and talking. I accept my vulnerabilities. And I continue to get stronger, even years later.

In my new life, it takes an absolute and deliberate commitment to be determined, tenacious, perseverant, relentless, and focused. And even if I'm not feeling particularly positive one day, I say I am. It's this assertive discipline that keeps negativity at a distance.

My daily challenge is to uphold and exemplify that grit and grace are elemental and essential for a successful recovery, no matter how steep the challenge is. I am grateful that I am here today to bring you, kind reader, on this journey of personal transformation.

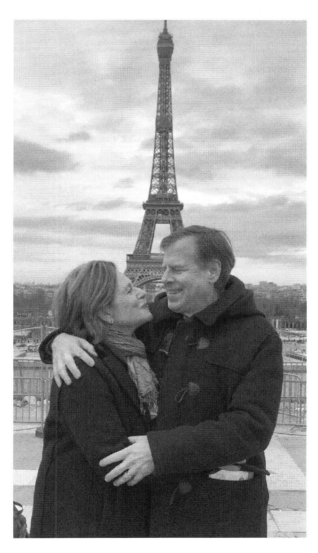

Pre-Pandemic Lockdown Trip to Paris with My Hero
(February 2020)

Acknowledgments

My Stroke in the Fast Lane would never be here without my mother, Betty Kogen, who saved my life and possibly many others driving on I-95 that Easter Sunday morning. My heart overflows with love, now and forever, for all you have given me, Mom.

To Janie Parks and Joe Manna, my Good Samaritans: You give us all hope in humankind.

To Michael Kogen, I am deeply grateful for you being such a caring and loving big brother. You made me feel so protected when you slept over in the guest area of the ICU one night. And the photos you had the wherewithal to take in the hospital are an integral part of this book.

To Pamela Kogen Morandi, my sister, I am forever grateful for your ongoing love and encouragement. Michael Morandi and Rebecca Kogen also played a big part in my recovery. Michael, I still have the email you sent to me: "Your recovery is an inspiration to us all and a testament to your character and determination. You came back to life during my faith's celebration of the resurrection, which will be indelibly etched in my mind whenever I celebrate Easter in the years to come. We are blessed by your presence in our lives."

To Corinne Brodnick and Morris Cohen, I love you both, and thank you for being so supportive along the way.

I am ever thankful to all my dear friends, near and far, here and overseas, for rooting for me. I heard you loud and clear! A special shout-out to Susie Tull. I am ever-grateful for our long friendship.

To the Sunday Night Gatherers, sincere appreciation for being my ongoing cheerleaders. I lived for our Sunday night Zoom calls during the pandemic, when we would assign someone to be the leader of our weekly discussions on favorite buildings, poems, paintings, album covers, gardens, cocktail recipes, objects from home, songs, restaurants, museums, morning rituals, movies, our last outing before the March 2020 lockdown, and where we would like to travel first post-Covid. Those calls were a diversion from the news as death tolls mounted astonishingly to 500 in the U.S., then into the millions worldwide.

Along with my sister Pamela and brother-in-law Michael, the SNG-ers include Laurence Waltman, Joseph Lembo, Mary Davis, Palmer Davis, Amy Godine, Jack Nicholson, Jill LeVine, Andrew Schwartz, Francesco Pardo, Bob Lane, Peg Harris, Sherwin Harris, Dru DeSantis, and Donna Placido.

To dear Jen Hammerstein, for always being there.

To Alice Moore for carrying on conversations and pretending nothing was wrong with me, especially when I ate soup. (Even though it went flying off my spoon, numerous times.)

Thank you to Ken Marsolais and Nancy Vick, co- producers of the documentary film, *The Bullish Farmer*. It was at lunch with Ken at The Outpost in Bedford, New York, that he encouraged me with this project and put me in touch with Stephanie Susnjara, writer/editor/content strategist. "Do you want me to call her now?" It was serendipitous that Stephanie was available to come down. We clicked immediately. It was she who was key to helping me organize my thoughts when I still wasn't able. Stephanie interviewed me for hours. The transcriptions of these interviews were a solid beginning to *My Stroke in the Fast Lane*.

I am also thankful for Susan Hodaro, memoir teacher extraordinaire, at the Hudson Valley Writers Center, along with the many writers in our workshops, for their early support.

To Paula Cappa, friend and editor, many thanks for all you do on behalf of the Pound Ridge Authors Society. Your steady friendship and sound advice are always much appreciated.

To Cynthia Wetzler for being such a great pal over the many years of our friendship.

Thank you to Daniel Snow and Mary Devine, who both helped me keep my head on straight.

Sincere thanks to Lisl Steiner, amazing photographer, documentarian, photojournalist, legend, goddess, and always my muse.

Extra love and appreciation to David Brodnick, Libby Mattern, my grandson Bowie Llewyn Brodnick, Annaclaire Brodnick, and Veneel Bhuthpathiraju.

And most of all, I'd like to honor my hero, Andrew Brodnick, whom I have known since tenth grade in high school. Endless gratitude for being my intrepid champion and loving companion. Your continued encouragement and nurturing give me the strength to say, *"I can do it!"*

Stroke and Drug Addiction Resources

CALL 911 IMMEDIATELY

Time is critical if someone is having a stroke.
The longer a stroke goes untreated, the more damage
can be done, possibly permanently, to the brain.

STROKE WARNING SIGNS:

THINK F. A. S. T. !!

- **Face drooping:** Is one side of the face drooping? Look at their eye, cheek, or lips to check for any unusual asymmetry or droopiness.

- **Arm weakness:** Is the person experiencing arm weakness? Ask them to raise both arms to shoulder height and check for one arm that seems lower than the other.

- **Slurred speech:** Is the person's speech slurred, or are they speaking in an unintelligible way?

- **Time to call 911:** Call 911 or your local emergency services. Be sure to tell them you think it's a stroke.

Resources

American Stroke Association (a division of American Heart Association)
Tel: 1-888-4-STROKE (1-888-478-7653)
Americanstroke.org

SAMHSA National Hotline (Substance Abuse and Mental Health Services Association)
Tel: 1-800-662-4357

About the Author

Bonni Brodnick is the author of *Pound Ridge Past*, now in its second edition. Formerly with *Glamour* and *House & Garden* magazines, Bonni has written scripts for Children's Television Workshop, was a weekly newspaper columnist, and was editor of two academic magazines. She is an award-winning communications specialist, a member of Pound Ridge Authors Society, and has a blog (bonnibrodnick.com). In addition, Bonni is an ambassador for the American Heart Association and a proud Stroke Survivor.

Made in the USA
Middletown, DE
05 November 2023

41752305R00090